Longevity Therapy

Dedication

This book is dedicated to my father, Lester G. Rothenberg, who allowed me to see that long-term care needs to include warm, creative, humanistic therapy to allow each elder to live to the fullest measure.

—Bobbie R. Graubarth-Szyller

Longevity Therapy

An Innovative Approach to
Nursing Home Care
of the Elderly

by

Bobbie R. Graubarth-Szyller, B.S., B.F.A.
Julianna D. Padgett, M.S.W., B.C.S.W.

with contributions by
Jules C. Weiss, M.A., A.T.R.

THE CHARLES PRESS, Publishers
Philadelphia

Longevity Therapy

Copyright © 1989 by The Charles Press, Publishers, Inc.

The Charles Press, Publishers
Post Office Box 15715
Philadelphia, Pennsylvania 19103

Library of Congress Cataloging-in-Publication Data

Graubarth-Szyller, Bobbie R.
    Longevity therapy : a positive approach to aging / Bobbie R.
  Graubarth-Szyller, Julianna D. Padgett, Jules C. Weiss.
       p.   cm.
    Bibliography: p.
    Includes index.
    ISBN 0-914783-30-0 (pbk.)
    1. Aged—Rehabilitation. 2. Nursing home care. 3. Geriatric nursing.
I. Padgett, Julianna D. II. Weiss, Jules C. III. Title.
    [DNLM: 1. Aging—psychology. 2. Homes for the Aged. 3. Nursing Homes.
4. Quality of Life. 5. Rehabilitation—in old age. WT 150 G774L]
RC954.G72 1989
362.6'1—dc 19
DNLM/DLC
for Library of Congress   89-821
                                    CIP

ISBN 0-914783-30-0

Editing, Design, and Production by Sanford Robinson
Composition by Cage Graphic Arts, Inc.
Photography by Jonathan S. Graubarth
Printed by Princeton University Press

5 4 3 2 1

Table of Contents

Table of Contents (Cont'd)

Table of Contents (Cont'd)

Acknowledgements

This manual emerged from more than ten years of exploring ideas and methods of promoting well-being in elders. These methods have been used with healthy elders in senior centers and with frail elderly in nursing homes. We have discussed these concepts with gerontological professionals and have presented them at conferences, workshops, in-service training for nurses, pharmacists, social workers, activities directors, and administrators.

In recent years this work has been supported by a grant from the Institute of Mental Hygiene, City of New Orleans. We thank them for their generous support. We hope the contribution of this manual will motivate more people to find new ways to touch the elders around them.

There are many people who have supported us in our work over these ten years, and it would be difficult to thank them all. But in particular we would like to say a special thanks to the residents and staff of the New Orleans Home and Rehabilitation Center, the Crescent City Health Care Center, and Willowwood Home for Jewish Aged, as well as members of the senior centers of New Orleans. Also we extend our gratitude to Julanne Haspel, Director of Jewish Family Service, who made it so much easier for us to complete this project by giving friendship and encouragement in many ways.

Introduction

This book proposes a new, innovative plan for enhancing the lives of the elderly. It is based on our strong belief that old age can be a time of growth, vitality, and contentment, not a period of decline and wasting.

The establishment of nursing homes has been our society's response to the care of the elderly. Until the present era, elderly parents usually lived with their children and grandchildren under one roof; but times have changed and the extended family has all but disappeared. In addition, life expectancy has increased greatly in the past few decades, creating a sharp rise in the elderly population. It is estimated that more than 12% of the total population will soon be over 65 years of age. Regardless of sociological causes, the number of nursing home residents has grown enormously within a short time.

Because of this influx, nursing homes have been hard pressed to keep pace with the needs of their clients. For the most part, nursing homes are still perceived as "last stops" where old people sit in chairs hour after hour, staring off into space, doing nothing, saying nothing—just awaiting a welcome visitor, death. Although this morose picture may overstate the problem of institutional care, the fact is that many nursing homes continue to function as they did years ago, focusing only on the physical and not the emotional needs of the elderly.

We are convinced that new concepts and models of caregiving are desperately needed. The emphasis of nursing home care must be on meeting the emotional needs of the residents and on providing an environment for learning, living and growth. *The nursing home should serve as a center for living, not dying.* The methods and practices we utilize to achieve these objectives form the core of this book.

The material presented here is meant primarily for the professional staff of nursing homes but should be of no less value to those who work with the elderly in other settings. Nurses, social workers, activity directors, administrators and aides in nursing homes will find the material adaptable to their programs. Also, those who provide home health care—a vitally important, growing field—should be able to utilize the principles and practices described here in dealing with their clients.

The success of our program depends heavily on motivation and self-determination, not only on the client's part but also on the staff's. Without strong belief in your work, without chances to learn new skills and to see the impact of your contribution, health care and social service can be unmotivating, unfulfilling and draining. We believe that the staff and clients have many needs in common: both need support, encouragement, opportunities to explore potentials, and the chance to use all of their abilities.

Some may argue that the concepts and methods we propose are utopian and perhaps even unrealistic for most nursing homes. After all, many facilities find it difficult even to provide good physical care, let alone any other care. However, we believe that what may seen to be utopian care today will soon be the standard of care for all nursing homes. Moreover, our experience indicates that most nursing homes can readily adapt at least portions of our program within the framework of their existing operations.

We hope this book, based on our own experience with Longevity Therapy during the past 10 years, will serve to inspire the staff and, in turn, clients to examine their roles and determine how to get the most from life. Advances in the field of gerontology make these exciting times, with new concepts emerging from psychology, group work, movement therapy, and community development. The techniques of yoga, meditation, New Games, touch, counseling, and group leadership illustrate principles that can be applied in your workplace. We urge you to explore the ideas presented in this book. Above all we would emphasize the importance of starting with the premise that change is indeed possible regardless of age, and that each of us should pursue the opportunity to change, particularly to change within ourselves.

The development of the concept of Longevity Therapy and its evolution will be of interest to many readers, especially those involved with designing similar programs. To this end, we have included the senior author's (BGS) personal reflections of how she started and became involved in this program.

Section One

Concepts of
Longevity Therapy

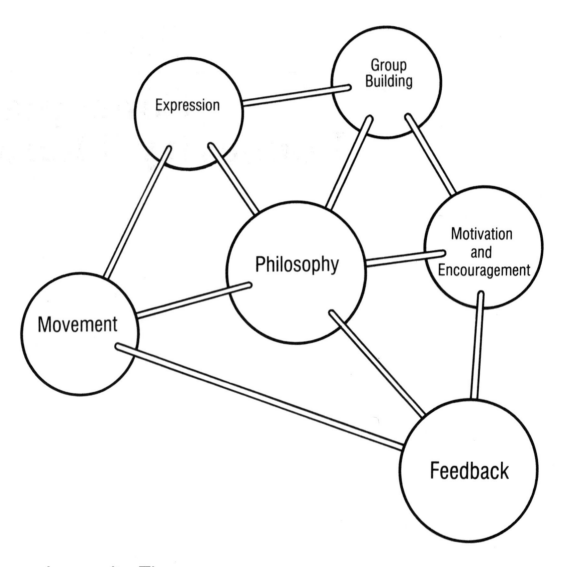

Longevity Therapy:
The Six Basic Components

Longevity Therapy

What is Longevity Therapy?

The term Longevity Therapy requires explanation at the very outset. It does not, alas, refer to a method for achieving old age or extending the life span. Rather, Longevity Therapy is an organized program designed to make old age a vital and fulfilling segment of life, by resisting the physical, emotional and social decay that so often characterize this period. Put differently, Longevity Therapy is based on the belief that aging need not be associated with decline; old age can be a time of awakening—the start of a fresh life from within. This book describes the various ways and means that we use to help elders, especially those in nursing homes, to accomplish this objective.

An Overview

Before we go on to the specific details of the program, let us first present an overview for orientation purposes.

In a broad sense, Longevity Therapy is a motivational program meant to offer elders an opportunity to make positive changes in their emotional and physical being and to experience the pleasure of change and the expression of feelings. The program is built around six basic components: **Philosophy, Movement, Motivation, Expression, Group Building** and **Feedback.** As you will see, the program uses group work as the primary format for integrating these fundamental components. However, the ultimate success of the plan depends on the group leader's ability and sensitivity in incorporating these elements into a productive system for each person in the group. We are convinced that the dynamics of a creative, caring group experience can beneficially effect physical, social and emotional change. But even without a group, the same principles can still be used in working with individuals.

In practice, the program involves a series of diverse experiences which are designed first to help participants maintain physical and mental flexibility. Beyond this initial objective, the components of the system are used to encourage self-expression, self-assertiveness and self-confidence. The methods used to accomplish these goals include body movement with music; yoga; breathing exercises; group poetry; relaxation techniques; creative play; and art—among dozens of others. Although many of these techniques may seem unusual and even beyond the scope and ability of nursing home residents, our experience indicates quite the opposite: elders are able with proper motivation to participate in many (or most) of these activities, even though the extent of their participation may vary greatly. That the resident is willing to try these activities is in itself a major step toward success.

Some Benefits of the Program

These group activities bring about many positive changes in the individual participants, including:

☐ strengthening the individual's emotional makeup through the pleasure derived from movement, sensory stimulation and social interaction
☐ developing, strengthening and reinforcing psychological and motor abilities, leading to reduced dependence and increased self-reliance
☐ making elders aware of physical tensions and learning ways to release these tensions and relax, thereby promoting better sleep
☐ recognizing inner feelings and how to respond to them in healthy ways (stress management can help, among other things, in controlling high blood pressure)
☐ promoting a sense of being psychologically competent and personally effective
☐ helping others in the group, thereby building and maintaining one's own coping skills
☐ facilitating friendship and intimacy within a group setting.

Each group activity is designed to build on the individual's strength, accepting the person's limitations and respecting his ability to make decisions about attendance and participation.

The program is usually conducted by two group leaders. One leader models and demonstrates an activity while the other is working with clients individually. The leaders must be able to recognize cues and to respond to small changes, encouraging each participant to do as much as possible within his or her physical capacities.

The Leader's Role

The leader's role is described fully in subsequent sections, but it is important at the beginning to affirm that the leader recognizes and agrees with the following fundamental premises of Longevity Therapy:

☐ Growth can occur at any age.

☐ Later years can be used as a time for self-development.

☐ An elder must accept personal responsibility in participating in his or her health care.

☐ Emotional expression through arts and physical activity promotes growth and helps maintain personal identity.

☐ Breathing and relaxation techniques are essential to health.

☐ Every person is unique and has a unique story to tell.

In the following pages, each component of the program is discussed in greater detail. Later we will give you more information about how to combine these components into a whole greater than the sum of its parts.

Philosophy

"There is a purpose to old age, a future to be fulfilled. The first part of life is for learning, the second for service and the last is time for oneself."

—*Rinpoche Tarthang Tolka*

In the 1950s, the renowned psychologist, Erik Erikson, developed a theory of the "Eight Stages of Man." He described old age or maturity as a unique stage of psychological development. Erikson said that the task of maturity, the last stage of life, is to resolve the conflict between "ego integrity vs. despair." This means, can you look back on your life and feel good about it? Can you maintain your self-esteem in spite of multiple losses of health, income, relationships? Or will you despair?

Carl Jung, the pioneering Swiss psychoanalyst, understood that there is a profound opportunity available to persons in the last stage of life. Jung, one of the greatest psychological and humanistic thinkers of our time, wrote:

> *But it is a great mistake to suppose that the meaning of life is exhausted with the period of youth and expansion;...the afternoon of life is just as full of meaning as the morning, only its meaning and purpose are different.*

Eastern cultures give support to both Erikson's and Jung's vision of the third stage of life. Later years, in Eastern culture, were deemed to be the time for individual growth and development. Instead of being a time of stagnation, these years were spent in contemplation and self-discovery. For example, the ideal age in Eastern culture to begin to practice yoga was 53, the age which marks the passage into a new stage of life.

These philosophies and traditions point to the need for old people to be released from the expectation that they perform as they did earlier in life. The new task of gaining "ego integrity" requires contemplation, self-discovery and self-awareness. The challenge therefore is to move from the outward thrust of youth to the discovery of the inner self. For a person to reach ego integrity in the last years of life takes acceptance and love of self. For many people, however, a sense of despair about themselves begins to set in early in life. Their true happy self—the unique child that was born into this world—has suffered hurt, abuse, disappointment. The child that was shining like a diamond is now, in old age, hidden under layers of emotional protection, admonitions and self-doubt.

We believe that the diamond is still there. If that diamond can begin to be uncovered, the person has a better chance to maintain integrity. The diamond is the fundamental truth about that human being; it does not change over time despite a lifetime of hurt. How can an elder begin to uncover the inner diamond? The answer is support. Wherever the older person is—in a hospital, a nursing home, or at home—the individual needs support. The elder needs help, as we all do, to move into a feeling of self-acceptance. We all need affirmation, encouragement, challenge, guidance, stimulation and permission to explore new feelings. When emotional and mental growth are supported, the physical body has its best chance to maintain flexibility and strength and vice versa. Longevity Therapy offers this support. It provides elders with an opportunity to maintain their mental, emotional and physical well-being.

Individual Responsibility

Fundamental to the success of Longevity Therapy is the need for preserving an individual's responsibility for self. Erikson's theory of development implies that every stage of life brings with it a responsibility for choice. To the last day, all of us *choose* how to live our lives. We need to continually remind ourselves of our choices— far too easily we get caught in a sense of having our lives dictated by outside forces instead of by our own internal decision and desires.

For an elder the choices appear to get increasingly limited. Loss of mobility, of income, of emotional support, take a tremendous toll on each person's psyche and emotional strength. But the fact of our individual responsibility never changes. As long as we have the ability to make decisions, we have responsibility to care for ourselves, in whatever way we can.*

Robert Butler, the psychiatrist, suggested that many older persons

---

* *We recognize that life-support systems and technology do deprive some elders of the choices to have their life naturally end.*

come to face a point of "responsible dependency." This is a person's ability to make a realistic evaluation of his need for help from others, and to accept that help with dignity and cooperativeness. The choice to become dependent in certain area is a responsible choice when one also makes the choice to be independent in as many ways as possible. This process means that a person has come to understand the limits of what is possible, can choose what to oppose and what to accept, when to struggle and when to allow. *This is one of the most important psychological tasks older people must face.*

Always remember:

- ☐ Growth can occur at any age.
- ☐ Taking responsibility for body, mind and spirit is everybody's right.
- ☐ One has an obligation to take action on his or her own behalf.
- ☐ Later years can be time for self-development.
- ☐ Respect but don't hold on to the past.
- ☐ You don't stop playing because you grow old, you grow old because you stop playing.

As staff, our role is to help elders assess their "ability to respond" and to help and encourage them to exercise that responsibility. What happens when a person makes choices? Acts responsibly on his own behalf? That person feels involved, active and aware of the possibility for change.

Movement

Disabled elderly persons suffer greatly from the social, environmental, physical, and psychological complications caused by inactivity. Diminished activity takes a toll on the biological functioning of their bodies, their feelings of well-being, their usefulness to themselves and others, and on their ability to function in the future and remain independent.

Well-designed movement therapy, coupled with proper breathing exercises, allows the elder to gradually increase awareness of the body, the emotions, and how they are linked together. Adding an emotional dimension to range-of-motion exercises allows people to respond with their total selves.

In the movement program, we follow certain guidelines:

☐ With encouragement, elders can regain movement and reverse some of the impact of inactivity.
☐ Tight muscles, in a sense, hold tension. Moving and relaxing the muscles releases tensions and has a positive effect upon mood and energy.
☐ Choose appropriate movement exercises with appropriate pacing.
☐ Each exercise is done with specific awareness of the body part that is being moved.
☐ Visualization helps to reinforce movement and the effects of the movement.
☐ Each movement has its own rhythm, and incorporating breathing is important to make the movement more effective.
☐ After each movement (flexing, tensing, bending, twisting, etc.), equal time is given to relax the muscles involved.

Longevity Therapy incorporates several movement systems into the program. These are summarized here and then described in detail in the next section on Methods:

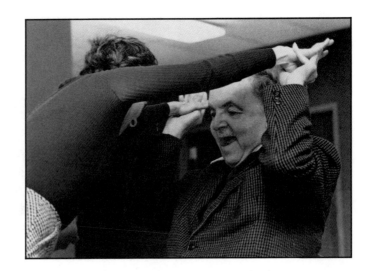

Bio-energetics incorporates an emotional component to the exercises by helping one to discover some personal insights. Here an elder is releasing "the weight of the world" from his shoulders.

Yoga

The application of yoga principles teaches the body to move in rhythm with breathing. When breathing correctly, movement is easier; one learns to release tensions slowly, without force. By awakening a rhythm in the body, yoga allows movement to flow with less hesitation. With yoga's gentle stretching movements, elders begin to feel changes in their bodies. Most people experience increased flexibility and a new surge of energy. These changes, however minor, are motivating to the elder and encourage continuing participation.

Bio-energetics

The term *bio-energetics* refers broadly to changes in energy within the body. Practically speaking, it provides a way of understanding how much energy a person has, how he uses his energy, and how he responds to life's situations. Several exercise techniques affect energy levels by incorporating an emotional component into the program. These exercises use movements associated with an emotional feeling, allowing the elder to discover some personal insight and at the same time to experience improved muscle tone and a release from tension. Bio-energetics teaches that we utilize energy most effectively when it can be freely translated into movement and expression. For example, a depressed person can rarely lift himself out of a depression by "thinking positive thoughts." This is in part because his energy level is depressed. When the energy level is raised (through techniques such as deep breathing, relaxation, expression), the person can emerge from the depressed state more easily. The energetic processes of the body are related to the state of aliveness of the body. The more alive one is, the more energy one has, and vice versa.

Tai Chi

Tai Chi is an ancient Chinese system of movement that incorporates swaying and slow dancing, encouraging the sense of balance that is so vital to an older person. Tai Chi trains one's body to become aware of support from the ground. The image of a balanced scale is used to help a person visualize how shifting weight and slow movement can lead to a sense of balance and control that is possible when we allow the ground to truly support us. Tai Chi encourages the pantomime, make-believe element of slow motion, bringing grace and imagination into an elder's life.

Toning/ Singing

The use of sound is an important group activity that is used to build unity as well as give an opportunity for expression. Sound produces internal movement that can be coordinated with external movement for healthy, easy, and often joyful activity.

Tapping

Exercises like tapping are encouraged for gaining awareness of circulation in our bodies. The elder can immediately feel a sensation on his skin from the gentle tapping technique, which is self-administered. The wrists are held loosely while the tapping movement of the hand is applied to different parts of the body. This causes an awakening sensation, along with relief of tension. Tapping can be combined with music and rhythm.

Play

We all need encouragement to be un-selfconscious while we explore new feelings and movements. Play is one of the best ways to rediscover some of the positive attitudes that come from being un-selfconscious. Play also increases one's desire to move and to laugh, a form of internal movement. New Games is a form of play which is safe and non-competitive; everyone can win, particularly in achieving an increased range of motion. Parachute play performed by a senior automatically allows repeated range-of-motion exercise that would make a physical therapist envious, and the use of props such as over-sized balloons increases enjoyment.

Massage

Massage supplies tactile awareness. It can be performed individually or within the group. Elders are encouraged to massage hands frequently as part of "homework." Back and shoulder massage is frequently done in groups to supply touching, an activity that is missed by people in this age category. The response to massage/

touching is often overwhelming; everyone needs to be touched. The release and appreciation are very noticeable. Massage can be incorporated into our regular contact with the residents. Remember that touching is vitally important, and use it often.

There are of course many variations of these methods, as well as other forms of physical activity. These are discussed in Section Two, Methods of Longevity Therapy.

Teach residents that daily movement serves to improve the physical condition, stimulate energy, and bring body and mind into harmony. This should be a constant theme of the program.

Motivation

Motivation is a critical factor in the success of Longevity Therapy groups. The Longevity Therapy staff constantly motivate the group and the individual participants by creating an atmosphere of caring, ease, and acceptance. Without motivation, the spirit of self-discovery and self-awareness would be greatly lessened.

Motivation begins with "where the client is." Each participant comes to the group with a certain energy level, mood, body posture, attitude, and experience. These are what he or she brings to the group. This is "where the client is." With practice, the leader can learn to recognize quickly all of these gifts, and thus be able to recognize and encourage small changes and growing power within the individual.

The key to motivation is a paradox. When you motivate, do not try to change the person. Instead, accept the person and all he or she brings to the group, both positive and negative. As you accept the person and *show* your acceptance, a trust relationship begins. Then you can begin to focus on a particular strength—something positive the participant has offered. This positive element or strength is then used to build and motivate other strengths.

In groups, here is how the process works. The leader:

1. observes the participant carefully
2. assesses the participant's strengths
3. reaches out with eye contact, touch, and a sincere statement
4. observes how the participant responds
5. expands the response.

Usually, the participant will follow the leader's expanded suggestion. For example, the participant whose level of participation is low: The only strength he offers may be simply his presence in the group. The leader uses eye contact, touch, and sincere expression to communicate "I am so glad you came to the group. I hope you will enjoy yourself." Then the leader continues to use touch as a means of involving the participant throughout the session. At the next session, the leader may try to build on another recognized strength.

For other participants who seem to be working below their level of competence, modeling is a great motivator to connect the individual with his or her own abilities. For instance: in one group, a resident named John did not raise his arms very high in movement exercises. The leader approached him and said, "I saw you raise your hands, John, and I think you can easily reach up to mine." He did, and continued at a higher level through the exercise. The leader pointed out to the group, "You see how well John reaches, let's all reach up like John." With this, John raised his arms even higher. John was clearly motivated by serving as a model to the group.

With a withdrawn resident, you may cue into his desire to be needed—"Would you help by holding the ribbon? We need you in the circle." The resident usually will reach out and join in by helping to hold the ribbon.

There are many reasons that can motivate a person to take a first step. For instance, a participant can be motivated:

- ☐ to achieve an end result, such as greater flexibility or feeling better
- ☐ because he or she wants to be a leader among peers and contribute to the group
- ☐ by being reminded of a past successful experience
- ☐ because he wants to please the leader, other staff, or family
- ☐ because he wants to express himself as an individual
- ☐ as a response to emotional or philosophical concepts discussed in group which serve as stimuli.

The key, the magic, is *not to force change, but to explore the positive, no matter how small*. When you use something a person has created (a tone, a movement, a smile, or just his presence), that person usually feels more highly valued—"I am acceptable and I have something to give." *This* is when the magical connection begins to happen, and that magical connection can lead to greater self-awareness for the group member.

Expression

Many elders, as a result of longstanding cultural and social conditioning, are stifled in the expression of emotional, creative, and imaginative impulses. One function of the group is to create a safe, permissive environment where the resident may feel comfortable expressing "negative" as well as "positive" emotions. Recent medical research has documented how the suppression of emotions such as fear, hate and anger impair the body's normal functioning. The goal in working with elders is to encourage the vital flow of energy that may have been hindered by years of maintaining an emotional restraining pattern. We encourage expression of feelings such as grief, pain, loneliness, and anger because when an emotion is expressed, there can be a release of pain and suffering. Conscious expression of feeling can release pent-up emotional suffering and replace it with peacefulness and internal balance.

Another form of expression that we encourage is that of the imagination, the creative process. Care givers need to encourage the elder to regain access to and develop the imagination. Imaginative work or play is a kind of festivity that enables the resident to relate to that part of himself which is expansive, intuitive, creative, playful, and *non*-task oriented. It is self-generating, because sharing ideas and feelings offers new material for further exploration.

Many avenues are available for emotional expression, and it is here that staff needs to be open and responsive in order to create an arena for experiment. Activities such as poetry, creative play, New Games, role playing, and free-form movement are only some of the things that can be done to encourage vital flow of expression. In turn, expression can lead to a clearer understanding of one's self in a new environment, and to be creative with the resources available.

The expressive and creative process alows us to look at the world differently, expanding our opportunities and options.

Many methods are available to foster expression. Ideally, the goal is to combine the creative process with expression of feelings. As described in the following section on Methods, the main techniques used toward this end are:

☐ **Art** Drawing, painting, or other forms of art represent an excellent means of self-expression.
☐ **Poetry** Creating a group poem serves to recall and reinforce the past, especially happy memories for the participants.
☐ **Music** Sound is an effective method for promoting movement and visualization.
☐ Other activities, such as creative play, games, role playing and free-form movement. These techniques (along with many others) can be used to encourage a vital flow of expression.

Expression produces other benefits that may not be as apparent. For example, expression can lead to a clearer understanding of one's self and how to take care of one's self in a new environment, and how to be creative with available resources. In effect, the expressive and creative process allows us to look at our lives differently, expanding our opportunities and options.

Feedback

Feedback is another pivotal component of Longevity Therapy. Feedback mechanisms, seen at all stages of the program, are broadly defined as any verbal or nonverbal communication that allows the leader and participant to gain more information about each other. Increasing self-awareness in a supportive atmosphere is a major goal of Longevity Therapy.

Longevity Therapy feedback is designed to:

- ☐ help participant and staff continually interact about what is needed to become more aware of self
- ☐ be specific and descriptive of behavior
- ☐ be given in such a way that the participant can respond and act if he or she wishes
- ☐ be based on a foundation of trust
- ☐ emphasize the positive, healthy elements of the person
- ☐ recognize the importance of the small changes in an individual's life.

Feedback is the component that shifts the focus from the group process to the individual.

Feedback can be gained in Longevity Therapy in the following ways:

- ☐ **Assessment** Staff uses initial activities of each session to assess the mood of the group and to establish open communication within the group. Activities are planned (such as parachute play or "echo game") to allow physical and emotional expression by the participants.
- ☐ **Program Flexibility** Although every session is planned, staff are trained to be aware of feelings expressed by individuals and to respond with a more appropriate activity, if necessary, than the planned one. By doing so, staff members model a way to deal with feelings immediately and adapt to change.
- ☐ **Homework** To emphasize self-help and to strengthen continuity between sessions, each individual is asked to choose a movement

he would like to work on between groups. The selection is recorded and reports are asked for at the beginning of each session. Homework reports are not mandatory, but those individuals who do participate by expressing problems or successes can be further helped by the leaders and by the group.

☐ **"My Day"** This is a mechanism designed to help staff evaluate their own daily activities. Based on the belief that a person cannot help others change until he understands the process of change within his own life, "My Day" leads the staff through a review of a day. It helps the staff establish new goals and is a parallel to "homework" for the participant. A form used to evaluate daily activities is shown on the next page. This evaluation is meant for the staff, but occasionally it can serve to motivate and provide feedback to the elder himself.

Personal Daily Activity Evaluation

My Day

	Action	Feeling
Identify one "win"* you had today.		
Identify one instance of self-assertiveness** you used today.		
Identify one exercise you enjoyed today.		
A goal for tomorrow		

* **Win:** A goal that you successfully accomplished.
Self-assertiveness: Taking care of yourself by acknowledging and expressing your feelings and thoughts.

Group Building

Group Building means creating a healthy, supportive environment—a community. Often elders encounter a very disconnected environment and become disconnected from themselves and from their own wisdom. Over 50% of elders in nursing homes have no close family. We must therefore create alternative families. Group building fosters the idea of family, of reconnecting and understanding that each person's life matters. Living in a supportive community can heal wounds suffered from loss of social role and change of lifestyle that elders so often experience. With their newfound roles, lives of elders can regain quality and meaning. Community is powerful!

Group building means community, not only within the group, but extending throughout the entire institution. Community means connection, caring, sharing, and togetherness. Community is essential both for the staff and the clientele of an institution and for the development of the individual.

All of the techniques and philosophy discussed in this book concern how people learn to care for themselves. Working with groups has proven to be an important method and environment in which to teach the individual to accept responsibility for himself. Furthermore, group activities permit the members to learn to trust each other. In a nursing home, this trust helps promote sharing and socializing outside the group.

Learning the diverse new skills which comprise Longevity Therapy is a process that requires deliberate introduction and continuing reinforcement. It is often difficult for a person to learn how to express his feelings freely, or to be assertive, or to perform yoga or stretching exercises. In a group, residents learn that others have these problems and that members of the group share their feelings and will help them. To see others benefiting from these skills is a good way to begin to understand the value of those new skills and how they apply to one's own life. The chance for an individual to observe and explore at a comfortable pace is an important element of group process.

The key thought: *We exist and survive by building relationships — by sharing and caring for each other.* This is the basic purpose of group building.

Sharing experiences in a supportive environment creates a sense of community.

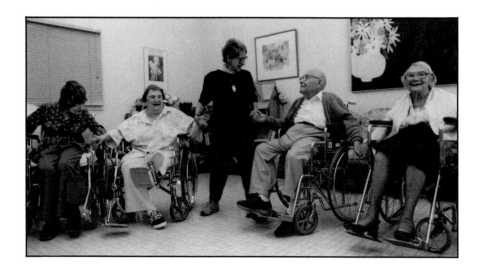

Section Two

Methods of Longevity Therapy

Introduction to Methods

This section focuses on many of the methods and activities we utilize in the Longevity Therapy Program.

Each of the activities is described using the same format:

Purpose

Who Can Participate

Size of Group

Materials

Description and Methods

Included in the description of some of the activities are Notes to the Leader and Case Histories.

Check-In

Purpose

Check-in is a form of introduction used to begin a group. Not only does it permit each person to be recognized as a member of the group, but it also provides the leader with an opportunity to assess each individual's mood at the time. Also, check-in sometimes serves to quickly uncover concerns of the participants.

Who Can Participate

Suitable for all residents. The specific form of the check-in may need to be varied according to the participant's ability to speak and similar factors, but individual recognition and attention should be given to every person as the check-in proceeds.

Size of Group

Include everyone in the group.

Check-in serves to make each individual feel unique. It is an important facet of Longevity Therapy. In this picture, the resident is identifying herself. Although she experienced a stroke, note how alert she appears.

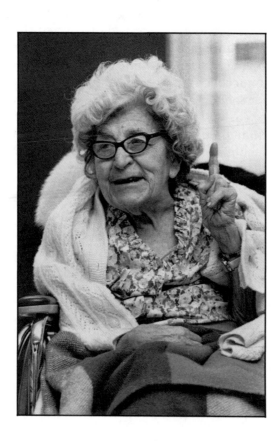

Materials

None required.

Description and Methods

Check-in can be almost any kind of greeting that elicits response of a feeling from the resident. The object is to make the participants comfortable in a group setting.

Simple word games can be used, such as the *Echo game:* The leader starts by introducing himself or herself with this rhyme:

Echo game, Echo game, _____ is my name.

The next person in the circle follows.

Another suggestion is to use the group-goal theme for the day and introduce it during check-in. If the theme, for example, is "taking care of one's self," ask each person to say his or her name and then tell "one thing I want to do for myself today." Some other typical themes: "one exercise I want to do today"; "I feel _____ today." This exercise can be combined with Echo game.

Case History

A woman in her mid-50's with Parkinson's disease responded to the "I feel _____ today" game with the word "frustrated." We encouraged her to elaborate and discovered that she wanted to eat in the dining room with the others but was afraid she would be too sloppy because of her disability. With the support of the group she approached the activities director, who contacted dining room personnel. They designed a space that would make it easier for her to eat with other residents. She now eats most of her meals in the dining room and is more content. The staff was unaware of her feelings until this little game was played. She had not mentioned it before.

Exercises In Bed

Purpose

Exercise has great value for all residents and should be encouraged repeatedly. Physical activity, no matter how brief, serves to reinforce the basic concept that each person needs to be responsible in some way for his own mind, body and spirit. Beginning with gentle movements in bed can be a motivating force for the rest of the day. Some of the benefits of these in-bed exercises are:

☐ encourages self-help
☐ allows the body to release muscle tension and stiffness that often develop overnight
☐ produces a stimulus that encourages the body to keep moving easily throughout the day
☐ focuses on a positive start to a new day.

Who Can Participate

All residents should try to exercise, no matter what their physical limitations may be. For residents who have little range of motion or who are bedridden, small micro-movements are very useful. The extent of activity will of course depend on the person's condition and physical ability.

Size of Group

Exercises can be taught in a small group and then practiced individually.

Materials

None required. (We have contemplated the use of a loudspeaker or closed-circuit in-house TV to encourage exercise in bed. In this way, nurses, aides and environmental staff could remind residents to exercise upon awakening.)

Description and Methods

Following are three different exercises that can be done in bed.

Stretching

Suggest to the group that they visualize a cat stretching, then stretch like a cat—extending both arms, both legs, separately, together and diagonally.

Active Motion

Instructions: Lie in bed and relax. Try to bring the right knee toward your chest. Use your hands to help. Take two deep breaths before the leg is raised and then exhale as the leg is returned to its normal position. Do the same with the left knee. Repeat the exercise five times with each leg. Go slowly.

Rocking

Instructions: Curl up like a baby and gently turn from side to side in an easy roll. Think of a baby relaxing and rock gently, moving the body from one side to the other.

Case History

Joe, a cerebral palsy patient with extremely limited range of motion as well as a fixed, frozen posture, was nevertheless able to accomplish a series of bed exercises. He intelligently adapted the exercises to his own level of ability. The ingenious workout he designed was remarkably effective and served to inspire the group when they became aware of it. (Because of his speech limitation, he had not told the group of his daily practice.)

Notes for the Leader

Although not every person can be motivated to perform bed exercises, it is important to continue encouraging the group. A few members will respond and they in turn will motivate others. The success of just a couple of residents often has a snowball effect and leads to a more positive attitude on the part of the entire group.

To begin the day with movement reinforces the basic concept that each person needs to be responsible in some way for his own body, mind, and spirit. Here the leader is modeling the Active Motion exercise.

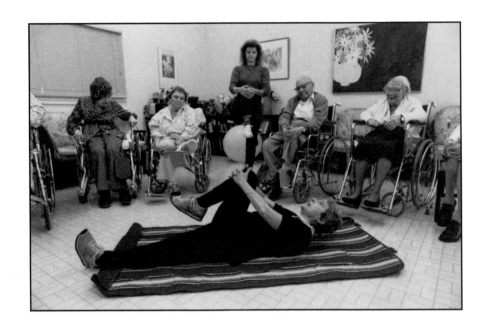

Breathing

Purpose

Breathing exercises will be beneficial to most people even if they can do them only occasionally. The person who is willing to practice these exercises will of course gain the most from them.

Who Can Participate

Residents with respiratory disease should have physician's approval before participating.

Size of Group

These exercises are best done in pairs, one-on-one, with an individual who has already learned them (and had some supervision from a leader) working with a novice.

Materials

To teach breathing, we often use a balloon to illustrate how one fills the abdomen with air and then slowly releases the breath from the top to the bottom of the abdomen last.

Description and Methods

First, get to know your normal breathing pattern. Sit comfortably, as straight as possible, with your eyes closed. Become aware of your inhalation, then your exhalation. Note how far down your breath goes. Upper chest? Lower abdomen? Is it more comfortable to inhale or to exhale? Spend a few minutes observing your normal breathing pattern.

Breathing and Feelings

Sit with your feet firmly on floor. Inhale and exhale through your nostrils, not through mouth. Then:

☐ Put one hand below your collar bone, near the top of the chest. Close your eyes and breathe slowly while you feel the upper chest; take 10 slow breaths. How does this feel? Register your feelings before you stop.
☐ Put one hand on your chest, close your eyes, breathe into upper chest only. Move only the part of the chest that your hand rests upon. Take 10 breaths. Register your feelings.
☐ Put one hand over your diaphragm, just below your rib cage.

Put the other hand on your chest. Now breathe into lower hand. Breathe in and out of your diaphragm. (Be patient, you know how to do this; you did it when you were young.) Take 10 breaths. Again, register your feelings.

☐ Now place your hand below your belly button three fingers below the navel. Try to draw breath into the lower abdomen so your chest and diaphragm don't move when you inhale, just the hand on the belly moves. Your chest will move only at the end of the breath. This means your lungs expand fully and fill completely with air. Twenty minutes a day will benefit, more is better. Better to practice on an empty stomach.

Under the leader's direction, this resident is practicing deep breathing.

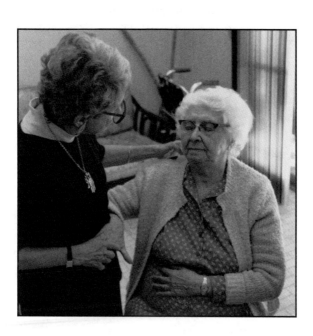

Notes for the Leader

The following suggestions may be helpful for the resident who is learning breathing techniques:

☐ If you are having trouble performing an exercise, try it while lying down on your back.
☐ Breathing into the lower abdomen is not easy. Be patient, keep trying. Work toward developing five to ten long, slow abdominal breaths. Imagine you are filling a long balloon inside your stomach: You have to inhale into the bottom first to fill the end of the balloon.
☐ When doing in-the-chest breathing you may feel upset or need to breathe rapidly to get enough air, or you may find it like the

way you breathe when stifling tears or feeling anxious. These feelings won't last; just notice them. . .and slowly relax your breathing.

☐ For the complete breath the benefits are many: It may be the most important exercise you do.

Directing the Breath

Begin to inhale, and as you do so, direct the breath

☐ to the abdomen, expanding it slightly
☐ to the middle rib cage
☐ to the upper lungs.

Begin to exhale, from the upper lungs

☐ to the middle ribs
☐ to the abdomen.

Use this rhythm:

☐ Inhale   4 beats
☐ Exhale   4 beats
☐ Hold   4 beats.

This is one round. Do six rounds or more. Once you are comfortable, you can prolong to six, eight, ten beats.

The 3-12-6 Breath

This is one round:

☐ Inhale very fully   3 beats
☐ Hold the breath   12 beats
☐ Exhale fully   6 beats

Do six rounds. Once you're comfortable, prolong the beats 4—16—8 and/or increase the number of rounds.

The Calming Breath

☐ Inhale and exhale once, then inhale fully.

- ☐ Retain the breath right below the collar-bone as long as you can, then calmly exhale.
- ☐ Rest a moment to normalize the breath, then inhale once.
- ☐ Exhale completely, contracting the abdomen, holding your breath out as long as you can, then
- ☐ Calmly and gently inhale.

Rest a moment; this is round one. As you practice you can hold the breath longer and enjoy the peaceful effect.

The "Ha!" Breath

This is another excellent release and is especially powerful if you add arm movements as if you are pushing the sound away with palms facing forward.

- ☐ Start with arms out in front of you at shoulder level, bringing them in toward the body as you inhale.
- ☐ As your arms come in, drop elbows at your sides so your hands are right in front of your shoulders.
- ☐ With a loud "Ha!" exhale as you push out with both hands. Move your right foot forward as you push. On the next push, move the left foot forward.

This is a very energizing exercise as well as an emotional release. *Remember:* Breathing takes practice! Relax and be patient with yourself. We all have a lifetime of poor breathing habits.

These residents are performing the "Ha!" breath.

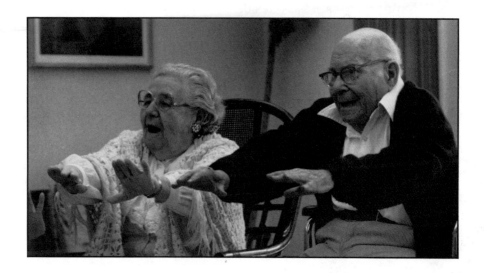

Yoga

Purpose

Yoga literally means *union*. It is a slow movement that unites the body and the breath. Yoga is based on slow, gentle stretching used with breathing to increase flexibility. This system of exercise, developed in India over a span of centuries, has important benefits:

☐ release of physical and mental tension
☐ improvement in posture
☐ relief of stiffness associated with arthritis and rheumatism
☐ redistribution of weight
☐ stimulation of circulation
☐ greater overall flexibility and muscle strength.

It is important for elders to maintain physical and mental flexibility—to keep moving, be active, and to adjust to the many changes and losses as one ages. Flexibility of body and mind helps keep elders from feeling "stuck." Yoga can be of great help in this regard. Also yoga rewards self-responsibility: an elder can *feel* its gentle benefits and thereby understand the basic premise that growth can occur at any age.

Who Can Participate

Some yoga exercises can be done by anyone. For bedridden residents, range-of-motion exercises can be incorporated with breathing exercises. For ambulatory residents it is beneficial to use mats and have them do yoga exercises on the floor.

Size of Group

The exercises can be done in groups of any size, or by individuals.

Materials

Soft instrumental music; mats for those who can lie on the floor.

Description and Methods

For those who have no idea of what basic yoga looks like, ask: "Can you picture how a cat or dog moves and stretches? Have you ever watched an animal wake up in the morning and enjoy a complete body stretch, top to bottom?"

34

Head and Neck Rotations

This exercise helps loosen the tight muscles of the neck and relieve tension. Pre-exercise instruction: Close your eyes, take three slow, deep breaths. Let your shoulders drop and relax. Both feet should be firmly planted on the floor or, if you're in a wheelchair, on the foot rests.

1. First, turn your head to the side as far as you can, comfortably. *Do not strain.* Notice how far you're turning your head by what you can see behind you.
2. Turn your head forward again. Close your eyes and check whether you feel relaxed. Your jaw should be loose, mouth slightly open.
3. Begin to roll your head from side to side very slowly, gently bending your neck toward your right shoulder.
4. Turn your head toward your right shoulder, slowly (10 seconds), then come back to an upright position.
5. Move head slowly (10 seconds) toward left shoulder.
6. Slowly let your head hang forward.

This completes one cycle.

Head and neck rotations help to relax tight neck muscles and relieve tension. Psychologically, keeping flexible is valuable in avoiding feeling "stuck."

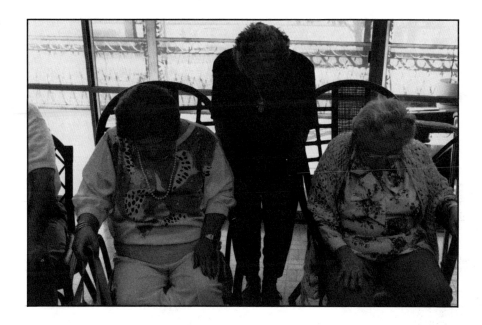

Whenever you feel resistance in moving your head, stop and "breathe into" the tense area of your neck until the tension melts. Then rotate head slowly back to center, taking up to a minute. Now rotate in opposite direction, paying close attention to the little spots of resistance or discomfort. Stop and "breathe into" any spot that seems tense.

Never do head rolls rapidly. When you are finished, turn your head as you did in the beginning of the exercise. Can you turn beyond the place you started today?

The kind of *awareness* that comes with slow movements and breathing cannot be found in fast exercises. The discovery of increased flexibility can be most encouraging to an elder and should help to motivate in an ongoing stretching, breathing yoga program. You can also do this exercise either seated or standing, with arms raised out to each side, parallel to the floor, palms up.

Eye exercises

1. Breathe deeply, feet planted, spine relaxed.
2. Open eyes wide, but do not strain.
3. Look straight down. Do not move your head, just your eyes.
4. Look to the right as far as possible.
5. Look to the left as far as possible.
6. Repeat steps 3 to 5 three times.
7. Roll your eyes in large circles slowly. Visualize the face of a clock and look at 12, 1, 2, 3, and so on. Breathe deeply as you go. Stretch and relax. Now reverse the direction, starting at 12, 11, 10, 9, and on through the cycle.
8. Close your eyes gently and "breathe into" the eye region. How do you feel?

Hand and Wrist Isolation

1. Take three deep breaths. Focus awareness on your hands.
2. Shake your hands as though they were floppy mops.
3. Move fingers as though typing or piano playing.
4. Make a fist, then let hand burst open with fingers straight.
5. Clap hands gently for one minute.
6. Rub hands together. When they feel warm, make a tight fist and then open fingers as wide as possible.

7. For wrists: Rotate both hands in the same direction, three times, then reverse three times in the opposite direction.
8. Bend your wrists so that your palms face forward, as if you were pushing a large object. You should feel this in the back of the wrist and the heel of the hand.

Other exercises

Shoulder rotations, arm circles, hip circles, knee rotations, ankle rotations, individual foot rotations can be done in the same careful manner with the goal of improving muscle tone and increasing flexibility. Learn the techniques well. Then tailor them to the individual's level of function and ability.

Yoga is an especially effective way to enhance movement in old age. It doesn't ignore safety and involves no equipment or other costs. Yoga offers invigorating exercise and mental discipline to an elder person in any condition. You start where you are and progess is easily recognized.

Notes for the Leader
In all of the exercises it is important that the spine be as straight as possible *(not rigid)* and that the resident's feet touch a hard surface, with weight distributed on both feet. Be sure the shoulders are relaxed (raised shoulders is *not* good posture). In explaining good posture, ask residents to imagine a golden thread suspended from the ceiling, connected to the top of the head and going down the spine and legs to the floor.

Encourage feedback. Most elders are able to recognize any improvement that yoga may produce and are of course encouraged by it.

Tai Chi

Purpose

This ancient Chinese form of movement is based on discovering the natural center of gravity in our bodies and using it to remain in balance. In Tai Chi we learn to feel the feet and the entire body supported by the ground in such a way that we gain new confidence in our movement.

Tai Chi movements are gentle, flowing, almost dreamlike. They serve to relax and loosen the muscles and joints, stimulate circulation, and build stability and internal strength. Tai Chi is practiced daily by millions of Chinese and an increasing number of North Americans and Europeans to maintain health of body and mind.

Each Tai Chi movement works on three common problems of elders:

- ☐ Loss of equilibrium
- ☐ Stiffness of joints and weakness of muscles
- ☐ Fear of falling and injury

Who Can Participate

Basic Tai Chi exercises can be adapted for most people, including those with very limited mobility. Keep in mind that balance can be achieved only when the individual feels supported and relaxed, regardless of body position. Even bed-ridden patients can be helped to feel more graceful and fluid in their simple movements. The keys are visualization of balance and proper support.

Size of Group

Best taught in a small group so that lots of individual attention can be given.

Materials

Large balloon and slow, quiet music (single flute or oriental sound).

Description and Methods

Introduce to the group the slow, dreamlike movements of Tai Chi. Explain that this movement form is practiced by Chinese elders to maintain health of the body and the mind. Movements are effortless and flowing and serve to relax and loosen the muscles and joints, to stimulate circulation, and to build stability and internal strength. It is most important for *balance*. The goal is to find your own center of gravity and to use the center to remain in balance, whatever you are doing.

Try this

Stand or sit with back straight, but not rigid. Imagine being suspended by a golden ribbon threading through each vertebra.

1. Shift weight slowly from foot to foot.
2. Breathe deeply and slowly. Imagine your nostrils are just below the navel. Breathe in and out from this area.
3. Now breathe in as you shift to one side and breathe out when you come to the center, the place of balance.
4. Raise arms in a circular attitude as if you were holding a very large balloon (we sometimes use large balloons as a prop to help achieve a circular movement). Continue shifting from side to side.

Tai Chi. Here, the leader is showing group members how to raise their arms as if holding a large balloon. Note leader in background demonstrating techniques with actual balloon.

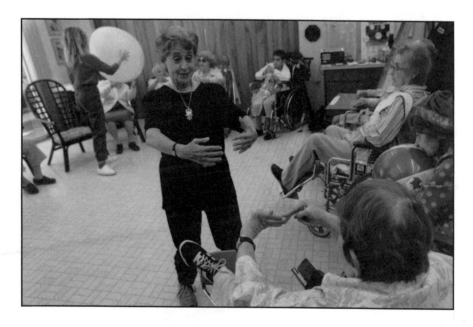

Try this

*Arm movements** For those who can stand: Place feet apart, shoulder width and feet parallel. Let arms hang relaxed at your sides. If you are in a wheelchair, sit up straight, be comfortable. Close your eyes and feel your center of gravity as follows. Imagine you are submerged in a miraculous fluid, thick, your favorite color.

*Adapted from Luce, G.G.: *Your Second Life*. New York, Delacorte Press, 1979.

You can breathe easily, but you will be moving as if under water.

1. Bend your knees and put weight into your feet. Slowly allow yourself to move arms and hands, letting them float in the thick fluid. Think of swimming slowly.
2. Gradually allow yourself to float in this translucent fluid; make movements slowly. Repeat until you feel relaxed. You may feel strangely silent during this experience.
3. Breathe into your center of gravity, approximately three inches below your navel.
4. Allow your arms to begin floating up in front of you, leaving wrists limp so your hands dangle. Imagine there are invisible strings pulling the arms up from the wrists. Let them rise, floating up to the shoulder very slowly. (This can be done in a wheelchair.) Be sure your feet are very heavy and your arms will float more easily.
5. Slowly let your hands float straight up, palms down, parallel to the floor. Keep your breathing relaxed.
6. Next, pull in your arms toward your shoulders, elbows bent, keeping your arms raised and close to your sides.
7. Bend your wrists and let your hands turn slowly so that your palms face forward.
8. Finally, let hands and arms *float* very slowly to your sides, as if they had to float through very thick, invisible liquid. Breathing is slow and relaxed.

The elder in this picture is performing Tai Chi arm movements. Note the calmly attentive quality of her facial expression.

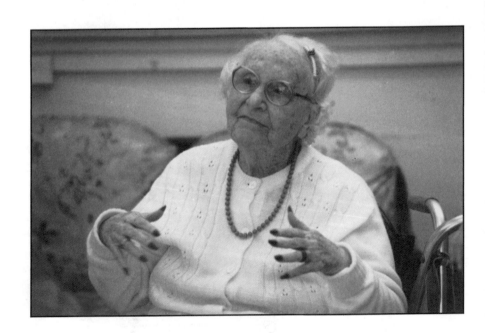

9. Breathe and feel your balance, your center. It may feel like you are floating through time; you may notice you have a greater sense of invulnerability. If you can feel your center as you walk or sit each day, you will feel less likely to fall. A very important benefit is that of standing or sitting alone, solidly, rooted to the ground, unable to be easily pushed or manipulated. You will be gaining greater balance and inner security.

10. Breathe in and out easily; these movements require slow, gentle breathing. Holding the breath would stop the floating feeling.

Notes for the Leader

These exercises work best when a resident can understand being "rooted" to the ground (the upper body is light; the weight is placed into the feet touching the floor). Tai Chi is never forced. The movement depends upon breathing and balance to achieve the floating, relaxed sensation.

Tai Chi exercise is excellent for elders. It is a true chance to experience relaxation in a positive, health-giving way. Describe this to residents as a movement that is very, very slow. Most older people respond well to the idea of "slow" movement. Make the most of this concept by suggesting that because older people understand "slow" more easily than younger people, this exercise is particularly designed for them. Let this be a light-hearted, fun discussion.

Case History

Mr. Fairfax, a 90-year-old, mentally alert man with hearing loss, felt a great deal of imbalance and had difficulty walking unaided. He became curious about Tai Chi. I worked with Mr. Fairfax, starting with deep breathing. He told me that, as a young man, he had been on a college crew team where he had learned the technique of deep breathing. Calling upon his experience, he relearned deep breathing quickly.

From breathing, we moved on to standing. At first, Mr. Fairfax could not stand alone, so I had him stand in front of a sturdy piece of furniture for safety. We worked on shifting his weight from foot to foot. I sugested he feel the floor through his feet, feeling a vital connection with the ground. Focusing on key ideas such as "I have my feet on the floor," and "I'm a grounded person," he began to feel safer as he took a few steps unaided. With practice, he gradually became more comfortable in his walking and less fearful about his balance, because he had been able to learn to shift his weight.

41

Meditation

Purpose

Throughout the world many people use meditation to achieve deep assurance, to find the light within themselves. The basis of meditation is relaxation, which is needed to reach an inner silence. This silence allows one to focus inward and leads to deeper understanding of the self. Observing our own life patterns and coming to accept ourselves are gifts of meditation.

At some level there is little difference between prayer, meditation, invocation, and other contemplative states. These are all states of being in which we are able to come to greater understanding of the reality of our existence and experience.

Broadly speaking, meditation takes two forms. The first stems from teachings focusing on the discovery of the nature of existence. The second concerns communication with the external or universal concept of the Divine, or God.

Meditation may be helpful in many ways. It calms, relaxes, promotes stillness, improves concentration, and, helps one to deal more effectively with physical and mental problems.

Who Can Participate

Meditation can be taught to all residents except those who are unable to remain quiet during the meditation time. Each person will find an aspect of meditation that is right for him.

Materials

Quiet background music may be beneficial.

Description and Methods

A basic relaxation technique should be used for 5 to 10 minutes. The object is to prepare the mind and body for meditation by stillness and quietness. Relaxation can be achieved as follows:

1. Sit in a comfortable position.
2. Relax your muscles and become still.
3. Breathe slowly, inhaling and exhaling smoothly.
4. Feel your nervous system become calm.
5. Relax the body; let the relaxation become deeper and deeper.

6. Notice the inner silence that comes with the body relaxed and still, while breathing slowly and regularly, and with the mind peaceful.
7. Enjoy the senses that become alive with inner silence.
8. Note the thoughts and feelings that arise, but do not hold onto them.
9. Let go of all thoughts gradually and remain this way for 5 to 10 minutes.
10. Accept yourself and accept your inner silence.

Observing our own life patterns and coming to accept ourselves are gifts of meditation.

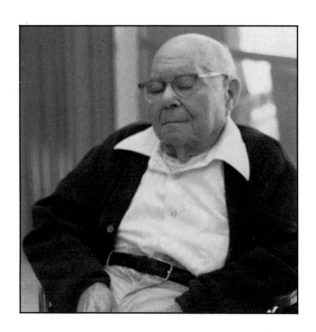

Notes for the Leader

Some thoughts about meditation and death: Psychologist Charles Garfield investigated attitudes of patients and their feelings about death and dying. His survey, *The Psychosocial Care of the Dying Patient,* showed that meditative experiences seem to lead patients toward a more positive attitude about dying. They had less fear and generally had more positive attitudes about death.

One central idea: The life of a human being can be understood as a process of spiritualization which reaches its climax with death. If a person can be guided past everyday problems, material concerns, pain, family difficulties, and some parts of the person can be extended beyond this "conditional reality," then he can feel free. He will be in unity with a greater whole, spacious and light. There is the sense that the spirit is strong and is able to carry on despite burdens. This feeling is what we want most of all for elders, and we believe it can be achieved most gracefully through meditation.

Relaxation

Purpose

Relaxation permits the body to function optimally. Through relaxation, tension and stress are released, thus allowing physical and mental energy to move easily.

Relaxation means, first, the absence of muscular tension. Some believe that relaxation is a state of collapse, but this is incorrect. Babies and cats look soft and flexible and are continually relaxed, yet neither is in a state of collapse. Although relaxed, both explore, are curious, and are able to express their feelings. When a baby is upset, it cries loudly. When a cat feels threatened, it responds visibly. The point is that anger, fear, loneliness, and other emotions can be expressed even in a relaxed state.

We know that much of the tension people feel comes from withholding of emotional expression. When we hold back tears, anger, clench our jaws, hide fear, we increase tension. The goal of relaxation, then, is not just to relax the muscles, but to relax the whole body and mind so that emotions can be truly expressed.

You can't relax with a busy mind! The mind affects the body's chemistry, which governs muscles, glands, and other organs. True relaxation will produce a clear thinking mind and benefit the way the body functions.

Who Can Participate

Almost anyone can be helped to relax. Simple massage, soothing music, and soft, restful words can reduce anxiety and fear for residents at all levels. With repeated exposure to the methods of relaxation, an individual will respond more and more rapidly to the suggestion to relax. Eventually, a person can generate a state of relaxation without any external suggestion.

Size of Group

Relaxation techniques are best taught in a small group, with the goal of encouraging individual practice outside the group.

Materials

Music on records or tapes can be very effective. Try very soft, instrumental music. Record stores often carry appropriate music in the "New Age" section. Health-food stores often stock cassette tapes that are useful for teaching relaxation techniques.

Description and Methods

Introduce the connection between mind and body with this thought: The key to relaxation is relaxation of the mind. With the mind's relaxation or quieting, we can become truly attuned to internal quiet and self-knowledge.

Autogenic Relaxation Techniques

This is a self-generated relaxation exercise in which carefully chosen phrases seem to allow release of tensions and help us enter a normal balanced state.

Instructions to Participants

☐ Get comfortable. Focus all your attention on your right arm, and say, "My right arm is heavy. . . .my right arm is heavy. . . . my right arm is heavy. . . .and I am at peace." Repeat this thought for 30-60 seconds and see how you feel.
☐ Then focus on the left arm, "My left arm is heavy. . . .my left arm is heavy. . . .my left arm is heavy. . . .and I am at peace."
☐ Make the same suggestion to the right leg, left leg, neck, shoulders, and chest. Notice what is happening and how relaxed you feel. (Many people have described the experience as one of healing, of unraveling the damages and tensions of the past.)

Notes for the Leader

We encourage group leaders to practice relaxation techniques themselves whenever possible, since a leader needs to experience firsthand the possibilities and benefits of this wellness technique. As a leader, you must feel good about yourself in order to be effective and stay balanced in your work.

Case History

A head nurse of a large rehabilitation institution had not had time recently to see what was going on in a Longevity Therapy group. On a day when she had been overly stressed, I invited her to join us, which I had done numerous times before. On this day, however, she accepted because she just had to slow down and regroup. That day we were planning to teach breathing and relaxation techniques. To allow participants to lie down, we had arranged to use the mats from the physical therapy department. The head nurse joined in the lying-down part of relaxation and the breathing exercises of the group. Soon she was more relaxed than the group had ever seen her, and several residents told her "Now you know what you've been missing!" Afterward she praised relaxation techniques and Longevity Therapy and commented to her staff about the fun she'd had in the group. Other nurses became more involved in Longevity Therapy after that.

Visualization

Purpose

Visualization (mental imagery) can be an effective method of relaxation and a powerful meditative tool to enhance all aspects of one's life. Mental imagery is something we use both consciously and unconsciously (for example, remembering scenes from the past, anticipating something in the future, or daydreaming). It can also be used to explore the unconscious mind, expand the individual's perspective on problems, rehearse unknown situations, and create a more positive attitude and self-image in order to promote self-healing. Visualization is, above all, an aid to restoring a sense of control over one's life, producing a more positive outlook.

When I first started doing yoga with groups in a nursing home, I needed a way to include the many severely-handicapped residents who attended. In order not to leave anyone out, I made suggestions based on what I had experienced from bio-feedback and relaxation, and techniques presented by Dr. Carl Symington in his book *Getting Well Again*. I encouraged everyone to be part of the yoga experience by saying "Those of you whose bodies have limited range of motion need to work just as hard—not by moving your bodies, but with your minds." At the outset, I asked handicapped residents to imagine or picture the yoga movement and do the movement by visualizing it. For those who questioned whether the mind can influence the body, I suggested: "Think of a nice, sour, juicy lemon. Now cut it in half. Picture the juice dripping; it is so juicy; now, take a bite out of the lemon." Immediately there were grimacing faces. This is a very graphic example to show the power of visualization as a lead-in to other methods.

—B.G.S.

Who Can Participate

Everyone who can and who will be attentive.

Size of Group

Any size.

Materials

Soft background music may be used.

Description and Methods

Slowly read aloud the autogenic relaxation exercise (*see* Relaxation). Then proceed with the following visualization suggestions:

Preparing for visualization

☐ Sit comfortably, eyes closed, feet flat on the floor, in a quiet room with soft lighting.

☐ Focus awareness on your breathing. Take a few deep breaths, and as you let out each breath, *mentally* say the world "relax."

☐ *Concentrate* on your face and feel any tension in the muscles around your eyes. Make a mental picture of this tension—it might be a rope tied in a knot or a clenched fist—and then mentally picture it loosening, becoming comfortable, like a limp rubber band.

☐ *Experience* the relaxation of muscles of your face and eyes. As tension disappears, feel a wave of relaxation spreading through your body.

☐ *Tense* the muscles of your face, especially around your eyes, squeezing them tightly like wringing out a wash cloth. Now, relax them and feel the relaxation spreading through your body.

☐ Move slowly down your body—jaw, neck, shoulder, back, upper and lower arms, hands, chest, abdomen, thighs, calves, ankles, feet—until every part of your body is more relaxed. For each part of the body, mentally picture the tension melting away, allowing relaxation.

Visualization 1

☐ Now, continue to picture yourself in pleasant, natural surroundings, wherever your mind's eye will allow you to go. It may be the beach, on a farm, or in a park, or you may be imagining a walk in the sunshine. Feel the sun or water's spray, or remember how this natural setting looked. Is it daytime or nighttime? Is it cold or hot? What are the sounds like? The odors?

☐ Continue for three minutes to picture yourself in this natural place.

☐ Let the muscles in your eyelids lighten up. Get ready to open your eyes and become aware of the room.

Visualization 2

☐ Observe yourself as you are, sitting in a chair. See the room around you. Notice the walls, decorations, floor, others in the room. Now focus your attention within. Close your eyes.

☐ Now visualize, in your mind's eye, the color red. Imagine a luscious, big, red tomato. See the red tomato gradually become larger. Allow the image to expand until everything in your vision is filled with a beautiful vibrant red. Gradually allow the image to fade.

☐ Take a few deep breaths and rest.

☐ In your imagination, focus on the color orange. See a ripe orange as vividly as you can. Let the image gradually become larger. Allow it to expand until everything you see is filled with a beautiful, vibrant orange. Now allow the image to fade away.

☐ In your imagination, focus on the color yellow. Imagine a large, bright yellow lemon. Allow the image to expand until everything you see is filled with a beautiful, vibrant yellow. Now allow the image to fade away.

☐ Now, see the color green. Imagine a big green tree with sunlit green leaves. Focus on the beautiful, sparkling green leaves. Let the image expand until everything you see is filled with sparkling green leaves. Allow the image to fade.

☐ Take several deep breaths and relax.

☐ Focus on the color blue. Imagine a clear, blue sky, the kind of sky you would see on a perfect, warm, spring day. Allow the image to fill your vision. Let it gradually fade.

☐ Picture yourself seated in your chair in this room, just as you are. Begin to gently, slowly, wiggle your toes, legs, fingers, arms. Take a slow, deliberate stretch, yawn, slowly coming back, ready to open your eyes.

Notes for the Leader

All directions must be spoken very slowly.

Remember, not everyone thinks visually. Some are more attuned to feeling. Suggest to the less visually-oriented people that they just *think* about the suggestions, rather than *see* them. *Use conceptual words interchangeably* ("feel" the color, "see" the color).

As the leader, it is important that you experience visualization firsthand. Put directions on an audio tape or have a friend read them to you.

A common problem during visualization exercises is the tendency for the mind to wander. This can be aggravated by medication, pain, or fear. Tell participants that when this happens, they should stop the process and ask themselves, "Why is my mind wandering?" Pursue this for a moment, then focus again on the exercises. You may want to photocopy the exercises and ask residents to practice in their rooms.

Occasionally a resident will belittle the exercises as mere "make believe." One way to respond is to make clear that visualization is not a method for self-deception, but for self-direction. (Be sure you're not unintentionally sending the message that the exercises are childish.)

Touch

Purpose

Touch is actual human contact: holding hands, a hug, hands on a shoulder or arm, combing someone's hair, helping someone shave. Touch is very important, particularly for residents in long-term nursing home facilities who may feel profoundly isolated.

Who Can Participate

Residents at every level. In skilled-care areas lie a multitude of elders who can benefit from just being touched. A gentle massage on hands, arms or feet can sometimes prove as beneficial as more complex forms of therapy, including drugs.

Materials

To facilitate hand massage, use lotion or massage oil.

Description and Methods

Hand massage

Hand self-massage Show the resident how to massage each hand: gently twist each finger starting at the base down to the nail, with just enough pressure to feel the difference. At the tip of finger, press the acupressure point (a sensitive area at the fleshy center of finger tip). Continue with massage by rubbing each palm, smoothing out muscles and rotating joints carefully.
Neighbor hand-massage Another form of exchange between residents is to encourage partner massage. Have the residents face each other and massage each other's hands.

Routine touching by staff

Touch residents when you visit, for example when giving out medication. Touch is a calming support that helps reduce fear and anxiety and communicates a sense of caring. Touch can sometimes reduce the need for pain medication.

Companion animals

Professionals are investigating the impact of having a pet on a person's physical and mental health. It has been suggested that a pet helps reduce stress, perhaps helping to lower blood pressure. The simple art of stroking and talking to an animal is pleasurable and provides companionship and a sense of intimacy that may otherwise be missing in a person's life. Pets can sometimes be borrowed from the SPCA. Some zoos have a program that brings pets to nursing homes on a regular basis. However, the best pet is a permanent mascot for the home. Regulations in federally subsidized housing assure that elderly and handicapped persons may keep pets. We hope this legislative trend will soon be extended to long-term care centers as well.

An additional thought: I used to bring my dog, Molly, an Irish setter, with me to the nursing home where I worked. I noticed that residents sometimes expressed their feelings about themselves through Molly, saying "Your dog looks very sad," meaning "I'm feeling pretty sad."

Notes for the Leader

Be sensitive to the resident who doesn't seem to welcome or enjoy touch. Respect his wishes, but keep the possibility alive. This attitude may change.

Breaking the barrier surrounding the isolated, inhibited, angry or docile client is a challenge. We have found that touch through massage can often help reach these individuals. As the other group leader is demonstrating one of the quieter techniques, I make contact with one of the residents through shoulder massage. The group members see me go from person to person and begin to look forward to their turn. Often I simply ask, "Would you like a soft massage or a harder touch?" This question supports elders in being aware of their preference and respects their choice. The brief, gentle contact tells the individual that he or she is cared for. I often feel the person's shoulders relax.

Does this divert the participant from the group? Only temporarily. The massage rarely lasts more than a minute.

Find the appropriate way to touch every group member and make a personal contact. Begin by greeting everyone as they come into the room. Be sensitive to individuals' personal requirements and whether they would respond more easily to a handshake or hug. Continue touching residents as you incorporate them into group activities, using the parachute, ribbon, balloons, or balls.

Remember how a newborn responds to touch? It is essential to hold an infant and touch it. Medical science confirms that a newborn can fail to thrive and even die without touch. Well, an elder needs this loving touch as much as a newborn! Elisabeth Kübler-Ross, Laura Huxley and others have suggested that care centers bring these two generations together so they can give to each other. Many nursing homes interact very successfully with nearby pre-schools or elementary schools. Children and elders can give each other a positive and loving experience.

Touch helps a person transcend pain, isolation, fear and loneliness. Build it into your groups as often as possible. I strongly suggest the leaders need to experience the joys of touching before leading it.

Self-administered massage is a pleasurable form of touch that enhances tactile awareness and promotes a sense of well-being.

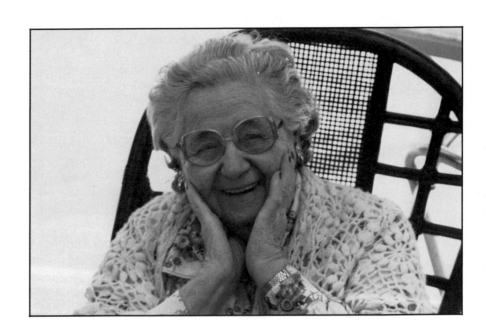

Case History

During a staff training session, one nurse reacted negatively when we talked about touching. When I started to demonstrate the methods of a shoulder massage, I sensed her pulling away. I quickly realized that she did not enjoy touching! Although I was hesitant to pursue it, I suggested that nurses who were bringing medications around in the cart try touch: massage on the shoulder area or hand. The next day she enthusiastically told me that she had tried the experiment. She had answered a request from a bed patient to bring in pain medication (it is not unusual for a patient to ring for medications when what she really wants is loving attention or a gesture involving touch) and when she came in and touched her first, making hand and eye contact for a few minutes, the client forgot to ask for the pills. Despite her earlier reservations, this nurse was pleased to discover that she could touch someone with such a successful and immediate result.

These elders are learning the technique of hand self-massage.

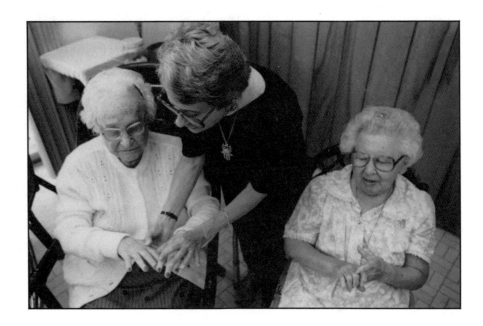

Self-Esteem

Purpose

Positive self-esteem is essential in maintaining control over one's life. Without self-esteem, elders soon drift to a state of helplessness and hopelessness, key manifestations of depression. Studies have shown that depression is one of the most pervasive problems in nursing homes and that institutions are often guilty of unwittingly fostering or accelerating depression by lack of attention to self-esteem. Indeed, a sense of esteem among residents is mandatory for health, independence and for living and dying with dignity.

One way to build or rebuild self-esteem is to encourage *choices*. Choices in a nursing home are as important as choices in other settings. The ability to make a choice reflects self-esteem and self-identity. It is important to encourage all residents to make meaningful choices whenever possible, and for the staff to promote this decision-making.

Typical choices that a resident should make:

☐ to be part of the nursing home community
☐ to be responsible and take care of one's self
☐ to learn when to oppose and when to accept suggestions of others
☐ to be assertive in asking for what is needed and to maintain personal integrity
☐ to live actively by not isolating oneself from others
☐ to reach out and do something for others; be active, not passive
☐ to live in the present, not holding on to the past but honoring it
☐ to spend some time each day on personal appearance: comb hair, accomplish good grooming and hygiene
☐ to feel as good about yourself as you can by expressing your concerns and finding solutions
☐ to decide to continue to make growth choices (self-actualization) as opposed to regression choices.

Size of Group

Minimum of four for the exercises described below.

Materials	None required.
Description and Methods	Self-esteem exercises are also described in Breathing, Encouraging Expression, Reminiscence and Assertiveness.

Breathing

A simple, direct way to build self-esteem is to breathe deeply. Deep breathing creates an awareness of the body, which aids in building self-esteem and a positive image. Another breathing method, the "Ha" breath (*see* Breathing), is used to gain an awareness of what one may need to feel a greater sense of self. Conceptually, much of emotional expression is to be aware and empty out the negative, thus creating space internally to rebuild the self-image.

Assertiveness

Being assertive also helps build self-esteem. It encourages the self, by asking for what is rightfully yours. An assertive resident has less risk of depression because of awareness of needs and how to meet them. Self-esteem is reduced greatly by subservience among elders who are too easily influenced by nursing home personnel. Subservient, servile behavior is a detriment to building a positive sense of self. This type of behavior should be discussed openly in a group, thus encouraging remarks that once spoken can be the basis of encouraging self-identity.

Mastery of Tasks

Performing useful tasks can effectively counter a lack of self-esteem. The task must be perceived to be worthwhile if it is used as a strategy for building and self-esteem. It is very important to break down the task into steps in order to ensure success. The elder should be involved in the choices, the planning, and the implementation of the task. This is time-consuming, but has its rewards in that the elders' input and abilities are reinforced.

The "I am" Game

This exercise is a powerful method to reinforce the individual's sense of personhood. It can be done with partners facing each other with the entire group standing in a circle. Go around the circle asking each resident to name (shout out) one of his or her roles in life. Responses such as "I am a mother, roommate, cook, lover of trees, enjoyer of food, reader, grandmother, worker, wife, husband," serve to identify the person as an entity and to reinforce self-esteem.

Giving to Others

This technique represents another way to build self-esteem. Giving can be done in many ways, such as visiting and feeding a bed patient, giving of the self through hand massage, or just listening and being actively responsive to others' needs. This type of reaching out to others needs to be encouraged. It has been said by gerontological visionaries that if every level helped the next level down, we would have fewer patients requiring skilled care. With this arrangement the skilled care patient feels loved, and the ambulatory resident finds a meaningful role in being needed.

Small Changes

At the end of a group session, suggest that every resident do one small thing differently that day and report what they did at the next group. The answers may be "I combed my hair before breakfast," "I visited with a new resident in his room," "I did deep breathing exercises when I had a pain in my back." That the resident was able to make a change in the daily pattern is a step in rebuilding a sense of self.

Notes for the Leader

Read the Reversal of Role Change Spiral (*see* Training) and be aware that you can be the Intervention. How do you do this? We find this sequence important:

1. Create an accepting, loving, safe environment.
2. Build a trust relationship.
3. Build vitality by breathing and movement exercises.
4. Encourage the release of pent-up emotions.
5. Then, add art, life review, poetry, reminiscence, and all the methods that focus on the uniqueness of the individual.

The ultimate goal of self-development in the aging population is *self-actualization*. A great humanistic psychologist, Abraham Maslow, developed a central theme that life offers much greater potential for happiness than most of us realize. His coined term, self-actualization, describes those people who have most fully developed their human potential. Maslow believed that we cannot reach our full potential until we have lived many years—until we have become old. Thus, aging and old age can be and ought to be a positive experience.

Positive self-esteem is essential to feel a sense of control over life.

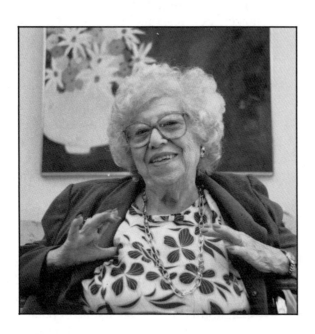

Case History

In discussing food with five relatively isolated, withdrawn residents, the leader asked about the foods they enjoyed cooking and preparing for others. The necessary ingredients were purchased the next day, and the group cooked their meals. An immediate transformation from withdrawn to very sure of their skills was evident. A hearing-impaired 85-year-old became the creator of a delicious New Orleans creole dish. She displayed more vitality than I had ever seen in her. A man with a deep depression told everyone his trout almondine couldn't be beat, and then he proved it.

By reaching into the past, these residents were able to tap into their positive self-image and experience self-esteem once again.

Self-Responsibility

Purpose

To give up taking care of oneself is to relinquish many of life's choices. Self-responsibility, therefore, wherever possible, is *mandatory*. Opportunities for using one's physical abilities and making emotional choices should be available to the resident at every level of care. If activities of daily living, such as dressing, can't be accomplished physically by an individual, verbal choices should be encouraged. The philosophy of *self-responsibility* is the main theme underlying all aspects of patient care. Accepting responsibility for one's self will allow a resident to function longer than one who simply depends on staff to meet all his or her needs. "Responsibility" implies the ability to respond.

Who Can Participate

Level of ability will determine the appropriate degree and forms of self-responsibility. For instance, the caring for plants described below may not be appropriate for a bed patient, but doing exercises in bed is quite appropriate. Motivating a resident toward performing a task that is appropriate and that could be accomplished with encouragement is very important. Emphasize the philosophy of self-responsibility and "responsible dependency" in every aspect of working with a group or an individual.

Size of Group

Any size.

Materials

A house plant.

Description and Methods

Try this

Bring a plant to a patient. An ideal plant would be one that is neither finicky, like an orchid, nor one that needs almost *no* care, like a cactus. Ask the resident to see that the plant gets sun, water and nurturing. Suggest "Just as you water and take care of your plant, so you need to take care of yourself." The message is that it is pointless to depend on anyone else for your own growth: for that you need to depend on yourself, and you need to give to yourself just as you give to the plant.

Encouragement and direction in caring for the plant are important. One study in a nursing home showed that those residents who were given a plant to take care of and taught how to be responsible for its growth nurtured the plant longer and more successfully than those residents in the control group who were given the plant without instructions.

Self-responsibility needs to be encouraged verbally, lovingly, and with conviction.

Case History

Emma T. was a permanent-placement resident in a nursing home. Her stroke had left her speech and right side impaired. She was a perfect candidate for group activity; I could see self-reliance in her expression. As a group we talked about responsibility, focused specifically on Emma, who was concerned about how much the stroke would limit her independence. Next time, when Emma came to the group, pushing her chair as a balancer, we marveled at her stamina and her determination not to give up taking care of herself. When she wanted to transfer to a chair in the circle, one of us stood by in case she needed help, but did not do anything for her, recognizing her need to find out if she could manage on her own. We watched this determined lady relearn skills that would keep her independent. Soon she allowed no one to help her do things she could do for herself. We pointed out to the group her attitude of self-responsibility, focusing on the specific actions she was taking to maintain herself. Emma became a model of self-responsibility, even taking in stride our praise of her efforts. She taught us the valuable lesson that nearly anything is possible with a positive attitude, action, and encouragement.

Notes for the Leader

How to encourage self-responsibility:

1. Talk about it; use the word "responsibility."
2. Suggest what choices are available.
3. Define problems clearly and outline specific steps for solving them.
4. Engage the resident in value clarification. (What is important to you?)
5. Ask for feedback, such as "How did you feel when you took an active part in dressing, feeding yourself, taking care of your room?"

Reminiscence

Purpose

Reminiscence and life recall is an effective process in working with elders. The process involves a review of the past with an opportunity to generate memories of one's life. Since elderly people often remember the past more clearly than recent experiences, reminiscences and life-recall techniques can help bring the past into focus. Also reminiscence can help an elder accept his present, not by itself, but within the context of an entire life. Life review is also an important way to foster self-esteem and reinforce the "I am" in an elder.

Who Can Participate

This is an effective method for all elders and works well even with disoriented individuals. In the latter group the extent of brain damage may affect the ability of the individual to regain clarity and self-expression; however, different parts of the brain may compensate for those areas not functioning appropriately. By exploring the areas of unknown potential instead of only looking at the individual's limitations, new areas of development and well-being may be uncovered.

Size of Group

Reminiscence is excellent in a small group.

Materials

Art materials (for Art and Reminiscence).

Description and Methods

Priming the Memory Bank

This exercise, adapted from Jean Houston's *The Possible Human* (Los Angeles, Jeremy P. Tarcher, 1982), is meant to recall images and incidents from childhood, eliciting uncensored information stored in the brain and body. This type of reminiscence has a tonic-like quality. The memories of childhood are still available to the adult and the results can be invigorating.

Instructions: Sit with a partner, close your eyes, breathe in slowly and relax. One of you begins by asking, "Tell me about..." The other answers. The goal is to tell brief memories about the subject, not one long story. Typical questions might be, "Tell me about..."

☐ your nicest birthday party
☐ something your family served for special celebrations
☐ a school friend
☐ your favorite candy
☐ eating an ice cream cone

Usually the result is laughter but sometimes the memories are not so happy. Suggest that we need to accept all of our memories, both bad and good, just because they are a part of ourselves. After each person has had a chance to "tell" his memories, share the experience with the leader or the group.

Art and Reminiscence (*see* Art)

Begin a reminiscence session with a discussion of a common item all participants would have a remembrance of, such as their childhood home or a car they owned or places they visited.

After a brief discussion, ask each person to draw a picture, using felt-tip pens and 12″×24″ paper. The picture should depict the items or subjects mentioned in the reminiscence discussion. While the participants draw, ask them not to talk or interact but rather to concentrate on drawing or writing anything they can remember about the subject. Talking often diffuses and interrupts the concentration of the participants in their written or graphic expression.

After the drawings are completed, have the participants discuss, one at a time, their pictures and memories. In this discussion, focus first on the participants' past experiences, listening to what they say, and subtly comment to reaffirm what they said. Then, lead the discussion to related experiences and encourage the participants to free-associate and recall their more recent past or to remember their earlier days. Use this process to help create a frame of understanding of the past. Once this has been achieved, try to help each person connect his experiences in a step-by-step fashion that finally permits an understanding of his life today.

Reminiscence can benefit a broad range of people: those who can recall only certain past experiences; those who have considerable trouble recalling their more recent past; and those who need an understanding of how their various life experiences were integrated. The leader should help participants connect the pieces of their lives in a step-by-step fashion until their pasts become clear to them. At this point, they often begin to remember and understand who they are and where they came from, and feel a solid sense of self, related to past and present.

Notes for the Leader

To gain insight and create changes by the directed reminiscence process described here can take a few sessions, or only one session to achieve, depending on the individual and the circumstance. If possible, place no specific time limit on these groups but allow them to follow their natural course (usually running from 30 to 90 minutes.) With participants who have engaged in this type of group experience before, discuss with them other possible experiences they can have at this stage of life and the future.

If you want to use reminiscence as your group focus, plan to begin the session with some slow stretching and deep breathing exercises. Also, use breathing and movement as a short break in the middle of the session. This will help the residents relax and may allow the memories to flow more easily.

Reminiscence can help an elder to accept her life history and the present as parts of the life process.

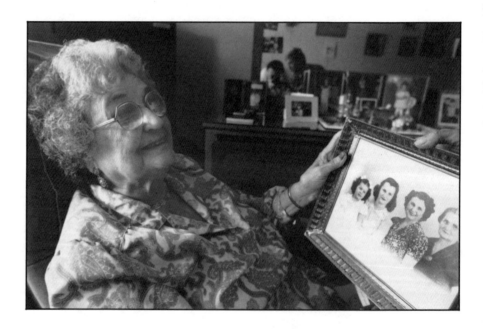

Mr. O. had been living in the home for a few months. He was a man in his early 70's who stood over 6 feet tall, usually unshaven, his thick grey hair uncombed. I often saw him in the hall and his usual comment was "Oh, I am hungry. Do you know when they serve food in this place?" Mr. O. (actually Dr. O.) used to be a dentist. He was diagnosed as having ASCVD (Arterioslerotic cerebrovascular disease). I introduced the Art Therapy session he attended by saying that we were going to draw something we loved in the past. Paper and felt-tip pens were passed out to the participants. Mr. O. didn't want to participate. The other group leader tried to motivate him, but he acted very stubbornly, claiming that he could not draw and would not try. I asked Mr. O. if the leader could give him a pen and help him by holding his writing hand and guiding it to enable him to write or draw what he would like to express. He agreed to this but it didn't work out too well. Finally, he wrote a few words very fast and drew some lines on his own; he appeared very agitated throughout the whole process.

Within fifteen to twenty minutes everyone had finished drawing. To begin the group discussion and break the ice in the group, I began talking about my own picture. I talked about how I love pizza and when I first discovered it as a child with my grandmother in Brooklyn, New York. I chose this line of discussion to show the group how my daily experiences and feelings as a child were intertwined with a deeply significant relationship with my family.

Next, I asked Mr. O. to talk about his picture. He said that he couldn't draw anything; however, he had written, "I am no good, I am no good at all." He read this over and over. In looking at his picture I noticed that he also wrote his name and drew a few lines. He appeared very depressed and frustrated. He then went on to say, "I can't draw, I can't do anything, I'm no good at all, I'm just stuck here." I nodded my head in agreement. I accepted his feelings. I accepted him. I commented that he must be feeling badly. He said, "Yes, I want to be with my sister. I hate it here." He then told me that his sister was at another nursing home and that is where he wants to go, to be with her. I commented that it sounds like he misses her very much and asked if he was very close to her throughout his life. He said, "Yes, very close," and he began to tell the group about his life. He began to talk clearly about his service during World War II as a medic, helping wounded soldiers in Europe. He then discussed coming back to the U.S., his life with his

65

family, and how his sister helped him financially and emotionally to get through dental school. He continued to talk about his career as a dentist, when he opened his first office, his second office; he even talked about some of his patients. For over 30 minutes Mr. O., a man who was usually confused and rambled about a variety of non-related subjects, was now clear in thought and expression and able to answer questions and communicate coherently his feelings and experiences of his life over the last forty years. This sudden improvement seemed like a miracle. Everyone in the group was stunned. No one had ever heard him talk so clearly, distinctly, and with appropriate affect and feeling. He proved able to recall much of his life vividly. It was as though he was a different man. He was sad in telling his story. He said he missed his sister. In conveying his stories and life experiences, he appeared to treasure the counting of his life. Throughout his discussion he seemed to be saying, "No, I am not a man who wasted his life like I am doing now in this nursing home. My life had meaning, purpose, fulfilling experiences, pleasure and joy which I cannot find in the nursing home; here, my life is a void." I seemed to have hit the right chord by letting him unwind his feelings and thoughts, and helping him recall and find meaning within the events of his life. He was able, with dignity, to express his sorrow and pain about where he is now. Possibly, his confusion did not come from organic brain impairment, but rather from the grief, sense of loss, and devastation he must have felt when he retired and entered a nursing home. In reflection, Mr. O's emotional and psychological pain created an anxious and uncomfortable tension within him that made it difficult for him to express his feelings without being rageful. To him, rage would have seemed inappropriate in the setting he lived in. So in order to diffuse his anger he became confused, locked into a pattern of maladaptive behavior, guilt, denial and confusion. Through the reminiscence group experience, Mr. O. was able to unleash his bound-up feelings and thoughts, expressing them to a group which accepted him for who he was.

After Mr. O. had talked, the group itself seemed to have awakened and opened its eyes. Even the nurse and nurses' aides who had been silent before began to talk more in the group sessions.

—J.C.W.

Reaching Up

Purpose

On the physical level reaching up is an exercise to produce energy and increase stamina and strength. It stretches the arms, shoulders, rib cage, and especially the chest muscles, which are commonly tightened with age. On a symbolic or metaphorical level, reaching up has richer meaning. The activity denotes moving upward, not being stagnant, not being afraid to try new things; but rather reaching to a higher level, beyond the body. Reaching up means reaching for what you want. *Above all, it is an action, and this is the secret of longevity—taking action on one's own behalf.*

Who Can Participate

Anyone with arm motion can "reach up." Residents whose arms are not functioning can "reach up" with their faces or eyes or toes. (Ask those residents to visualize their own "reaching up.") Of course, the range of motion may be restricted, but any upward movement is action. Look for indications of reaching up, however small, and immediately acknowledge them.

Size of Group

Any size.

Materials

Reaching up can be facilitated with balloons, sometimes with music as a motivator. (Choose your own music, for what *you* like will be the best choice, since you will enjoy leading it.) Another prop that may be used is a ribbon (*see* Ribbon/Circle).

Description and Methods

Reaching up is a metaphor as well as a movement. So we encourage the group to reach up and "reach for what you want." It's hard for a person to be depressed when his arms are reaching up. This can be demonstrated by modeling a posture of exhaustion and depression (when everything is down), and then lifting arms and body up and sensing how different you feel. Don't be afraid to use exaggeration in showing a depressed posture, exhausted, inverting the body, head hanging. Then model reaching up, arms overhead, hands as parallel as possible, palms facing each other or turned outward. Verbalize the entire exercise: how reaching up produces a different mood than does a downward movement, repeating that it is unusual to feel depressed when you're reaching up. Then lead "reaching up" with music.

You can also use a balloon, holding it over the resident's head to encourage them to reach up. While the two of you are holding the balloon, you can dance together, with the balloon between you—A Reaching-Up Balloon Dance! Then ask for feedback, and you will probably hear phrases such as "I feel alive," "energized." Reaching up can also be done with a ribbon (*see* Ribbon/Circle). Another suggestion is to use yoga with the posture of arms overhead, reaching and stretching with deep breathing.

Case History

Reaching up can be reaching for what you want. It is an action, and this is the key to longevity: taking action on one's own behalf.

Elise, an elderly woman who recently had a stroke, was admitted to the nursing home as a permanent placement. Her daughter felt that since her stroke Elise was unwilling to do what she could for herself. She became a Longevity Therapy group member. Since her stroke she had felt lowered self-esteem, but in the group we encouraged her and noticed each small improvement she made, thus helping to boost her self-esteem. She particularly liked the "reaching up" exercise. Elise learned yoga breathing and gentle, slow stretching. In art group she drew for the first time and expressed herself beautifully. During group work with movements, we encouraged Elise to make sounds, because she had yet to form words since her stroke.

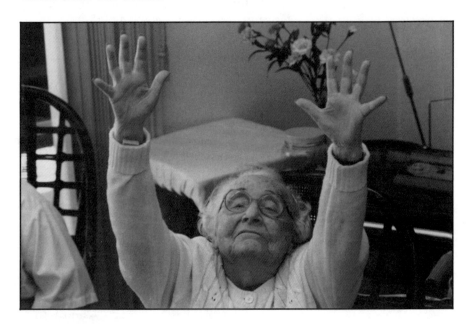

Group participation helped to counter her feelings of isolation and confusion. She now had many acceptable ways to express herself.

For her it was all non-verbal expression, but she was so involved in each activity that we could see and feel her growth and change as she learned new expressive methods—at age 75, with a recent history of stroke!

Elise was learning new ways to cope, to express, to enjoy her life. Elise was in Longevity Therapy for 17 months, after which she was able to leave the nursing home and live with her daughter.

Notes for the Leader

Longevity Therapy techniques and experiences are particularly successful for stroke clients, especially those with a speech problem. The non-language sounds and complete acceptance of whatever happens help relieve feelings of inadequacy.

Assertiveness

Purpose

Assertiveness is a way of communication that allows an individual to express feelings and opinions without violating another person's rights. Learning appropriate assertive behavior can help the nursing home resident avoid aggressive or passive communication—sometimes the only way people know how to handle the multiple frustrations of institutional life. In this sense, learning assertive communication is an important way to release tension and keep stress to a minimum, as well as to assure that elders speak up and express their opinions.

Who Can Participate

Those who are able to express an opinion or make choices should be encouraged to be assertive, especially if they exhibit aggressive or passive behavior. Assertive communication can be learned with practice and encouragement.

Size of Group

Teaching assertive behavior is best done in a small group, where members can learn from each other and practice in role-play demonstrations.

Materials

None required.

Description and Methods

1. The key to teaching assertive behavior is to help people understand their true feelings and how to communicate them effectively. Following is a general teaching plan, showing one example of what you could say:

    To communicate feelings effectively and assertively, it is essential to understand what your true feelings are about a situation or person. Understanding the truth about how you feel is extremely difficult; admitting these emotions is even harder. Take the time to talk about your feelings in the group or with someone else you can trust and who can give you an honest opinion about the situation you are experiencing.

2. Help each resident identify the assertive behaviors he or she already uses. Ask:

    Do you ask for what you need? Remember, it is important for

you to know your rights. Everyone has the right to self-expression. Open and honest communication, while not always available, is something you have a right to, and if you feel you are not being treated this way—speak up! Just because you are in a nursing home does not deprive you of your right to acknowledge and voice your feelings and opinions.

3. Help your clients learn the scope of assertive behavior, which can involve several different forms of communication, including:

- ☐ confrontation
- ☐ revealing and sharing emotions
- ☐ saying "no"
- ☐ saying "stop"
- ☐ putting your needs first
- ☐ negotiating
- ☐ requesting help
- ☐ requesting that you be left alone
- ☐ not taking responsibility for someone else's problem.

Learning assertive behavior can help the nursing home resident avoid aggressive or passive communication – sometimes the only way people know how to handle the many frustrations of institutional life.

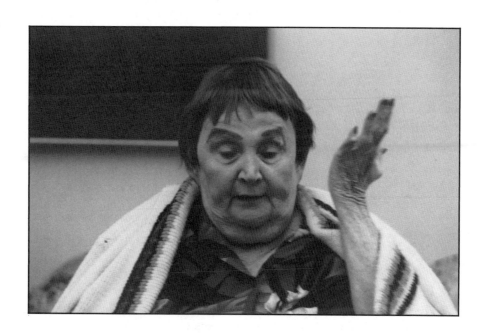

4. Discuss the difference between assertive and aggressive behavior and the meaning of passive-aggressive behavior.

Assertive behavior: expressing your feelings while respecting the rights of others

Aggressive behavior: dominating (controlling) a situation with disregard for the rights of others

Passive behavior: being submissive and not exerting one's rights.

Passive-aggressive behavior: using passiveness to control or manipulate situations at the expense of others.

5. Demonstrate and practice methods of assertive behavior with the group. For example, tell them:

Communicate your feelings clearly, referring to yourself as "I," specifically to indicate *your own* feelings. For example, it is more assertive to say "I felt angry when you did not speak to me yesterday," than it is to say "You made me angry when you did not speak to me yesterday." (No one *makes* us angry. Anger is our response to a situation and our feelings, whatever they are, are O.K. to express.)

6. Help elders identify the fears and concerns they may have about being assertive, especially in a nursing home. Explain:

Remember, assertiveness means expressing your feelings while respecting the rights of others. Being assertive does not mean that you will necessarily get what you want. It does mean, however, that you have opened communication and that you have not suppressed your feelings. You have had your say. This is good.

Case History

A woman who was confined to a wheelchair was repeatedly pushed from one place to another, often not knowing where she was being taken. While discussing assertiveness as a group, we role-played this particular situation. The woman learned quickly to say "stop" when someone pushed her and realized that she had a right to ask, "Would you tell me where I am going?" She was tremendously proud of taking control over this part of her life. The word spread, and staff became more respectful of all wheelchair residents.

Notes for the Leader

When you are teaching residents assertiveness skills, also try to encourage the staff to learn the skills for themselves. In any case, be sure to alert the staff that the residents are practicing assertiveness skills. This is important for two reasons. First, the residents will require the help of the staff if their efforts are to succeed. Second, a newly assertive patient is apt to provoke undesirable reactions in an uninformed staff. To avoid these problems it is helpful if the staff comes to the group to express their support.

Assertiveness training, as mentioned, can help reduce the incidence of hostility, passive-aggressiveness, and negativity. These behaviors are well known in nursing homes and often make the work of the staff more difficult. It is to everyone's advantage for residents to communicate freely and assertively.

Assertive behavior should be practiced as often as possible in the group. Help the participants express feelings, make decisions, and take control as often as possible, especially within the group setting. Explain how these same skills apply outside the group.

By encouraging assertive behavior, the leader can help to create a happier setting for residents and staff alike.

Body Image

Purpose

To help the individual become aware of posture and how it affects self-esteem. Body image—how you feel about how you look—partly determines your posture and reflects how you feel about yourself. An erect posture and straight spine help one to feel in control of the body.

Who Can Participate

All levels. There is a way for everyone to improve self-image. Posturing is not just sitting up straight, but using body mechanics to the best of one's ability. If a resident is unable to sit straight, deep breathing techniques can be used to enhance self-image.

Size of Group

These exercises can be accomplished individually or in a group of any size.

Materials

All that is needed is a chair that is firm, not too soft! If the resident is in a wheelchair, adjust the foot rest so the resident's feet can connect to the floor, if possible. In any case, instill awareness of the concept "solid footing."

Description and Methods

The leader should demonstrate a frozen posture (tight, rigid, soldier-like, shoulders tense and raised); then a depressed posture (head bent down, shoulders slumped). In both cases the breath cannot flow freely because of the posture. The thought is that obstruction of air flow causes a decrease in energy and a loss of full vitality. Make sure residents see and understand this idea. Then ask them to model postures of "exhaustion," "depression," "4-star general." Encourage laughter during this posturing, but remember the goal of self-awareness. Next, demonstrate how to posture:

1. Feet should be firmly rooted to the floor.
2. Spine should be straight as possible but not rigid. Imagine a ribbon threaded through the vertebrae, holding them in alignment.
3. Lean from side to side to find mid-point of balance.
4. Expand the chest with a deep breath.
5. Hold neck straight, but not rigid.

6. Visualize yourself as a Raggedy Ann or Andy doll—relaxed but upright. Note the difference between rigid and relaxed. Feel how relaxation brings vitality.

Notes for the Leader

Immediate and visible bodily changes can be observed during role-playing with different postures. Because these body adjustments can be seen quickly and easily, this exercise can provide excellent feedback for both leader and resident. The leader can support the resident in recognizing his ability to change, which will instill a sense of accomplishment. After physical change is noted, ask questions about internal changes that may have occurred during this period: Can you move easier? Breathe easier? Typical responses are "I become exhausted when I'm slumped over, my breath is caught in my body." "I feel very depressed when my spine isn't straight." In contrast, after attaining good posture, remarks often go like this: "I'm not as tired, I feel lighter." "I feel O.K., I'm going to be all right."

Love Tapping

Purpose

Tapping is an effective technique to bring energy into a group experience and particularly to start a group session. "Love" tapping evokes pleasant, tingling sensations and may help to increase circulation. It is also a way to focus attention on all parts of the body, including areas that a resident may ignore because of how she perceives a disability.

Who Can Participate

Residents at all levels. Be sure to encourage any resident who has had a stroke to participate and to use the strong side of the body to tap the affected side. When time permits, the leader should assist if necessary.

Help those residents who cannot move either arm or hand. Tap the face gently and then one arm. Encourage self-care by asking them to continue by "visualizing" the tapping. Ask them to think about "tapping energy" into the other side and the rest of the body.

Size of Group

Tapping can be accomplished with a group of any size as long as attention can be given to the individual.

Materials

Any upbeat music. Consider what music makes you feel happy and energetic and use that. It is your enthusiasm and the joy you display that will make this "love" tapping exercise successful.

Description and Methods

Love tapping is gentle, rhythmic contact, using loose fingers on any part of the body. It is often used to start a session, because it makes individuals aware of their bodies and brings energy to the group. It is a form of self-massage.

Try this

Loosen your hands by shaking them gently, then gently tap the left shoulder loosely with right hand. The object is to lovingly tap energy into the shoulders, going down your arms inch by inch. Tap different areas of the body in a rhythmic way as the music plays on.

Encourage residents to keep up love tapping between group meetings, particularly when a body part is in need of "waking up" or is stiff or needs extra attention.

Tapping is an especially effective and useful method. It includes action, pleasure, musical content, body awareness, and allows for feedback to the leader. It can quickly build energy into a group.

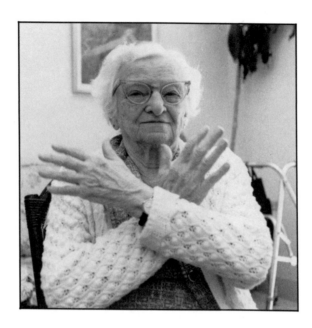

Encouraging Emotional Expression

Purpose

Residents should be encouraged to express their feelings, not only those of joy and pleasure, but also those of anger, grief, pain and loneliness. Emotional expression is a primary focus of Longevity Therapy because it is only when an emotion is *expressed* that there can be a release of pain. The underlying problem itself may not change dramatically, but one's *response* to the problem may change once it is expressed.

Some residents may be reluctant to "rock the boat" by expressing themselves because passive behavior tends to be encouraged in long-term settings. Lack of expression, however, can worsen many emotional problems and even cause new ones. Consciously expressing feelings, both negative and positive, can relieve the pressure of pent-up emotional suffering. Longevity Therapy groups can provide a safe environment for expression of these emotions. The ideal is that the entire institutional system would support the expression of feelings—that the system could even benefit from someone's "rocking the boat."

Who Can Participate

Although we refer to verbal expression in these exercises, it is also important to encourage speech-impaired residents to express emotions. Some stroke patients can benefit from these experiences, since many exercises include making sounds, non-verbal expression, and "body language."

Often a resident who is withdrawn or aloof will pull back from any show of emotions. Acceptance of this choice, coupled with supporting the resident in being more expressive, takes time and creative modeling by the leader.

Size of Group

No limit. All group members can participate.

Materials	Emotional expression can be accomplished anywhere with no props. All that is required is an artful leader who senses the unexpressed pain, sadness, fear, grief of the resident.
Notes for the Leader	I have used an elevator in a nursing home to allow for private expression such as crying and yelling out. The first time it wasn't planned. I was in the elevator bringing a resident to a Longevity Therapy group, when her emotional pain surfaced. I pushed the "stop" button and in effect gave her an isolated, soundproof space for letting out emotions that she didn't want others to see or hear. In fact, many residents (and the home) would benefit from a room designated for crying or yelling. Many nursing home staff members feel unequipped to deal with strong emotions and therefore do not encourage expression ("Don't cry, honey.") It would be healthier if the resident cried and expressed the feeling. Then it would be out of the body, no longer suppressed, and is less painful to deal with. A new resident in particular has a tremendous need to express emotions arising from all of the changes and losses inherent in making such a transition. (*see* Art, Poetry, Reminiscence, Feedback, Assertiveness, Toning and Check-In for further information and insight into emotional expression.)
Description and Methods	**The "Ha" Breath**

Suggest that everyone in the group inhale deeply, then exhale with the sound "Ha." This sound must come from deep in the belly; there is less strain there. Ask one member to tell what he would like to get rid of, something preventing him from feeling good today. Then demonstrate how to exhale with "Ha" while pushing your arms out, away from your body, metaphorically pushing out the negative feeling. This is an exhilarating exercise; usually people are smiling afterwards. (*See* Breathing, page 33.)

Emotional Chorus

Ask residents to "stand for" different emotional states (for example, angry, glad, joyous, silly, sullen) and form groups. Assign each emotion a specific sound: *Ah, Oh, Ugh.* In a playful spirit, direct residents in a chorus of sounds. Use good judgment about this exercise. When working well, it can lighten depression. Be sensitive, however, to individual needs. *Never* force participation.

Faces

This exercise encourages expression and is also important for maintaining flexibility, tone and circulation of face and neck muscles. Instruct participants: Close your eyes gently, take three deep breaths, relax, and imagine your face as a child. Feel your jaws, cheeks, nose, and forehead slowly relaxing.

- ☐ Close your eyes tightly, wrinkle your nose, and blow out your cheeks like a blowfish.
- ☐ Stick out your tongue and pop your eyes.
- ☐ Make face of a pouty little boy or girl.
- ☐ Squint and frown hard.
- ☐ Make the ugliest face you can.
- ☐ Make a face as if you just ate a lemon.
- ☐ Make a face of someone who is very angry, very sad, sleepy. Be delighted, aggressive, sullen, defiant, humble, frustrated, disappointed, make yourself laugh. Feel the difference in your face.

Notes for the Leader

Although these are playful exercises, it is important to keep in mind that the participants are *not* children. By giving them close attention, caring, touching, eye contact, listening, you will show them that you are not just playing games, but that you honor and encourage their truthful expression. Always ask for feedback, and if a resident needs more opportunity for expression, encourage that. On the other hand, a resident may be withdrawn and emotionally unable to express feelings at a given moment. Do not force this resident to participate. The time for expression has its individual timetable and can be encouraged but it should never be forced. Do create an environment, however, where people will feel safe.

These exercises are most effective when you are able both to have fun and to maintain a careful awareness of emotional cues.

As you become more sensitive to how residents can be approached, you can help other staff members to be more sensitive and respectful of residents' adult emotions. Staff should strive to avoid calling the residents names like "honey," which can convey a patronizing attitude. In doing so, the staff can better address the real needs of the residents as they begin to see them more clearly as individual personalities.

Motivation and emotional expression are closely linked. People who need to be motivated often don't see that certain limitations are self-imposed. They feel

- ☐ stuck in one place
- ☐ powerless
- ☐ without options.

They need to

- ☐ be able to see options
- ☐ be given achievable goals
- ☐ get rewards
- ☐ feel a sense of control.

The person who helps must

- ☐ be trusted and be worthy of trust
- ☐ believe that change is possible.

Toning

Purpose

Toning is a method of exploring our emotional range by means of sound produced in our own bodies. This technique of using internal vibration is mentioned in the ancient texts of several cultures and is one of the oldest methods for combatting pain and promoting relaxation. Toning has been reintroduced into the therapeutic setting by Laurel Keyes, author of *Toning, The Creative Power of the Voice.* Keyes says, "Beneath the words [we speak] are vibrations of the tone upon which they travel." She suggests that it is the tone of the voice which truly gives form to the ideas in our minds. We use toning when we sing a lullaby to soothe a baby's cry, and we also use toning in our speech. "As we speak, so do we live, inviting hostility or fulfillment and love." In these toning exercises, each individual expresses a sound that describes his emotional feeling.

Who Can Participate

Anyone capable of making sounds can participate. Toning is particularly good for stroke patients, who may have difficulty speaking, but who can make sounds.

As a speech pathologist working in the area of stroke rehabilitation, it has been my observation that Longevity Therapy has proven to be quite valuable and of added benefit to the communicatively impaired individual's speech and language therapy program. It has been noted to often indirectly enhance the progress made in therapy and allow for a means of carry-over outside the structured therapy session.

Longevity Therapy provides an opportunity for expression whether in a verbal or non-verbal manner. It helps to alleviate the feeling of isolation often felt as a result of a communication impairment due to stroke. Often the individuals who cannot utter words, can utter sounds and in doing so, participate in a sharing and expressive experience. Longevity Therapy helps to break down the "silence barrier."

—Allison M. Ewing
Speech Pathologist, M.A.T., CCC

Materials	None required.
Description and Methods	To begin, ask the group to groan. After that expression of sound, tell them you will be talking about toning and that anyone who can groan can tone. (You are making the connection for them.) Talk about the natural sounds of the body. Ask what the sounds are— groan, sigh, cry, laugh, scream. Suggest that until we were about five years old, that is how we probably responded to the feelings of the body; that toning allowed the free expression of sounds and of emotion. After that age, the natural sounds of the body were not as easily accepted. Many people, including parents, teachers, and other authority figures, taught us to control our expression, our sounds. As a result, most of us have a very narrow range of acceptable expression of sound. Toning helps in releasing these restrictive patterns and exploring the entire range of emotional expression through sound.

Groaning

Instructions: Keep your spine erect with feet several inches apart. Stretch both arms high, then let them drop back, with the shoulders swinging on the spine as a cross bar balances on top of a T. Then relax arms at your sides (if standing) or on your lap (if seated). Close the eyes, relax the jaw, teeth slightly parted. Let the body groan and feel the groan down in your feet and deeply throughout your body. Encourage continuing groaning, always starting with low groans. Let the *body* groan as long as it likes. One may think he has nothing to groan about, but it is surprising how the hurts, physical and emotional, will surface.

You may suggest to the resident that he do this tone in private until he is comfortable with the expression of feelings that may come forth.

Tell the resident: "Let your mind be still and just watch." After groaning, an audible deep sigh may be released, indicating that the body/voice is satisfied. Ask how a sigh feels (a sense of relief that something has been accomplished.)

During toning, let the body be free and let the voice be free. *This freedom is the most important factor in toning.*

Suggest toning be done upon awakening to set a positive pattern for the day.

Toning for Others

Think of the name of someone you wish to send love or healing thoughts. Toning is a way of sharing one's self with another person and can be given like a gift.

The Toning Scale

Use the notes of the "C" scale. "C" is first. Explain that it signifies *purification*. "E" is second. Significance: *healing* and *gratitude*. "G" is third. it signifies *acceptance that healing is started*.

One way of toning for others is to make three syllables of the person's name and tone the syllables using the musical notes C, E, G—moving up the scale:

> C is for purification
> E is for healing and gratitude
> G is for acceptance

The group can tone each member's name. Ask who would like his name toned and see the hands pop up!

Try this

An American Indian chant: "Hi-ya, Hi-ya, Hi-ya, HI." Repeat the chant until the group shows signs of slowing down. This, we have found, is a group favorite and can be used with the story of an old American Indian man, who used this chant on a two-hour trip. He got on the bus with cold symptoms—nose and ears all stopped up— and by repeating this chant softly, he opened up his nasal passages and sinuses by the end of the ride. This is a motivating story, and an excellent example of the use of toning in a case of physical symptoms.

Stomping can be added to the chant. Ambulatory residents can stomp, march and chant on tone; seated residents can stomp in place while chanting. You may want to demonstrate the toning first and then add the stomping.

Toning for Pain

Relief of pain is sometimes noted with toning. Method: Tone as low as the voice can reach, slowly raising the pitch (the way a siren sounds). One will find that there is a tone which seems to resonate with the pain and relieve tension. Every pain seems to have companion tone, and by pulsating that tone softly for as long as it feels good (fifteen minutes is optimal, if possible), the pain can be relieved. Toning is an escape valve for the pain, much like an inner sonar massage.

Notes for the Leader

This new method may cause some people to question its relevance to a therapeutic group experience. I, too, was skeptical when I first read about toning, so I invited a guest whose practice of toning and self-healing was respected to demonstrate the method. I watched a Longevity Therapy group follow her suggestions by sound, humming, groaning, reasonating their own tones into a guided experience. After this experience, the group asked for more toning exercises. They enjoyed the Indian chant best of all—it incorporates playfulness, release, and is almost hypnotic. But beyond the release and pleasure is the underlying concept that you can do a lot for yourself, first by believing in self-responsibility, then taking the action it requires, and seeing the belief system at work in the action. It is important that you, the leader, try this on your own, for example while driving to work. I practice everything first, and when it has become part of my belief system and my practice, then I can truly share. Toning is one of those wonderful, joyous alternatives.

—B.G.-S.

Music

To be in music is to be in meditation. Music is food for the soul.
                                 —The Orange Book

Purpose

Music is used in group settings and with individuals as a motivational technique and to elicit expression with the body and voice. Some benefits of music are as follows:

☐ encourages movement and improves coordination
☐ provides an opportunity to let go of tension and pain and move to a higher level of interaction
☐ allows the listener to leave everyday concerns and focus his awareness on the sound. That process creates a meditative state which fosters relaxation and reduces stress.
☐ creates micro-movement (below the level of muscular movement) within the body. Some believe that this movement stimulates the lymphatic system and other body systems, in a beneficial way.
☐ inspires joyful emotions that may stimulate release of certain chemicals (endorphins) in the body, which in turn promote a sense of well-being.

Who Can Participate

Because it affects us emotionally as well as physically, music is useful for all groups and individuals. The rhythm of music can be an essential factor in helping people respond at a nonverbal level, while promoting reconditioning of motor functions, voice control and self-expression.

Size of Group

Music can be used with individuals and with groups. It is often more fun to do music exercises in groups, especially rhythm exercises, but they can also be used with individuals.

Materials

Records, tapes, a tape recorder with a good speaker, rhythm sticks, musical instruments. (Records can usually be borrowed from the public library.) Don't forget that music groups and other entertainers often volunteer their time in nursing homes; their service generates good feelings.

The selection of music to be played depends on the activity being performed. Some of our personal choices are:

☐ For relaxation, Steven Halpern, *Zodiac Suite*
☐ For movement of joints, "Golden Slippers"
☐ For love tapping, Dave Brubeck, "Rotterdam Blues" on *We're All Together Again*
☐ For stimulating movement, with upbeat, strong rhythm: Dave Brubeck, "Sweet Georgia Brown"
☐ For movement to words: Papa Celestin, "Down by the Riverside"

Description and Methods

Music to Increase Sensory Perception

Play classical or contemplative sounds such as "Rhapsody in Blue" by Gershwin or "Zodiac Suite" by Steven Halpern. Ask the group to relax (*see* Relaxation, page 45), then play music for 5 to 10 minutes or until group gets restless. Be sure to "clown" as you suggest to the group that they try to listen through their feet. Then ask:

☐ How does music make you feel? Alive? Tired? Blue? Joyous? Peppy? Sleepy?
☐ What color does the music suggest?
☐ What did you see through your mind's eye?
☐ Did you feel the sounds? Through your ears? Through your eyes?

Use all senses and cross over from one sense to the other, with such terms as "feel" (kinesthetic), "hear" (auditory), and "through your eyes" (Visual) to create expansion of sensory perception.

Music to Create Imagery

Play "Inside," by Paul Horn, flutist (or a similar meditative sound). Ask the group to listen to the sounds and see, feel, hear the music and try to form a picture:

☐ Is it being played in the daytime or at night?
☐ What colors did you feel or see when you heard the music?
☐ What mood were you in when you heard it (calm, agitated, happy, angry)?
☐ What else did you see, feel, hear?
☐ Where was it being played?
☐ Were there people involved in the sound?
☐ Was nature a part of the scene (sky, water, field, mountains, sun, snow)?

Keeping Rhythm

Clap hands to a steady beat, either softly or loudly. (The expression of loud sounds can help release frustration in a socially acceptable way.) Sticks can be used for beating rhythm. A supply of sticks can be made by the residents, using ½-inch dowels which are sanded and painted. Or you can buy ready-made rhythm sticks in music stores.

Notes for the Leader

Using music is like having two extra group leaders to help. It also stimulates the staff. Remember not to use background music if it interferes with foreground sounds. Avoid very high or very low sounds with hearing-impaired clients, especially while you are talking.

Case History

Sometimes music is extremely personal, and what works for one resident may not work for another. For example, in trying to motivate Mrs. K., a German-born elder, to exercise her arm as part of a rehabilitation program, we tried all sorts of music to encourage movement. She resisted all suggestions of exercise. Finally, we put on a Strauss waltz. Mrs. K. responded promptly and began moving her arm.

Song

Purpose	Song is an excellent method to encourage expression. It also serves to increase lung expansion and breath control, to say nothing of being pleasurable to all. As a method of expression, song (and music) can

- ☐ enhance self-esteem, self-confidence and self-awareness
- ☐ increase social skills through interacting with neighbors while singing together
- ☐ increase the strength of the voice
- ☐ improve circulation and muscle tone of the upper body
- ☐ provide opportunities for a creative experience.

Who Can Participate

All residents should be encouraged to participate. Song is much easier than speech for some stroke patients. Don't be surprised when previously silent residents burst forth in song once they are part of a group.

Size of Group

Any size.

Materials

All that is needed is a tape recorder, a variety of tapes, and your willingness to be a lead singer who sings loudly.

Description and Methods

Use such songs as "Listen, Listen, Listen," and "From You I Receive" to increase awareness of community. These songs are excellent ways to sensitize the residents to group living, discouraging isolation and encouraging giving to others. We often use them as an ending song.

Singing is an outward-directed activity that promotes group enjoyment and group bonding. To teach a song, recite the words three times and then sing the melody. Next, play the tape with the residents listening. Then have everyone join in and repeat it as long as is appropriate. Ask for volunteers to tell what the lyrics mean to them. Then repeat the song. The song is often sung with more enthusiasm the last time.

You can also have the words of the song written out on cue cards in large letters.

Poetry

Purpose

Poetry, based on the use of images, helps the individual use the mind's creative capacities (located, for most people, in the right hemisphere of the brain). The play of words and images focuses on a person's intuitive self. Poetry is a wonderful means to encourage an elder to express a potential that is rarely tapped in a long-term environment.

Who Can Participate

Anyone who has the ability to respond to images and express feeling (the responses can be non-verbal).

Size of Group

Five to fifteen residents in a group.

Materials

Tape recorder, music tapes, pad and pen.

Description and Methods

One goal of poetry in a group is to create a "group poem." To do this, elicit immediate impressions and responses from each participant. Everyone's words are included and everyone is encouraged to contribute, even if it is only an audible sigh. Even the most "far-out" phrase will work in creating a group poem. Write the lines down as they are spoken and compose the poem right in the group. You and the participants will be delighted and touched by the beauty that can emerge from this exercise.

To create a group poem, ask the residents to express a simple thought or happening from the past, such as:

☐ The funniest time I can remember
☐ A trip with the family
☐ Something you never told anyone until now
☐ Bright yellow love
☐ Tell us where you aren't (evokes birthplace, humor, lifestages)
☐ What kind of tree do you feel like?

Write down the responses and comments of the group to construct a poem of phrases.

Another method is to listen to music and record participants' responses.

This is a poem a nursing home group wrote after listening to Paul Horn's music, "Inside."

> I wail my notes up to the dome
> Echo pause
> Echo. . .echo
> Sound, effects, blue sound
> Lament for the beauty that is gone
> Lament for the beauty that is

Notes for the Leader

Poetry helps express feelings of the past and allows the past to become a living reality today. In *I Never Told Anybody,* author Kenneth Koch has compiled writings of people in a nursing home. Reading some of this material to the poetry group can be stimulating and helpful. Another author, Mark Kaminsky, wrote *The Uses of Reminiscence.* These books will expand the options available to you in opening the doors to the richness of memory.

Art

Purpose

Art, all too often regarded as merely a children's pastime, can be a significant mode of intervention and a powerful communicative tool in working with adults and the elderly. Although some adults may think that creating artwork is childish because it reminds them of their youth, or regard it as a simplistic activity owing to their lack of training and experience, art can be a vital form of personal expression for everyone.

Art is one dynamic way to deeper understanding of one's self.

Using simple techniques, even the most timid will be able to make some type of drawing. Those who resist the process because "I can't draw a straight line" will be assured that the art process is not a competition, not a matter of talent, but rather a way of being in touch with the rich inner resources of each individual. *Creativity is ageless.* According to R. Butler & M. Lewis, authors of *Aging and Mental Health,* "Creativity in old age means having the opportunity to attend to parts of ourselves that we never had time or energy or a chance to develop earlier, to be honest, in a new way, with less invested."

There are three types of art experiences health-care professionals can offer to participants: crafts, expressive arts, and skill-learning activities. At different levels of participant competence, these three types of art activities may interweave. For example, a simple craft can become a skill-learning activity as the individual develops competence in creating the craft object. Or an expressive arts creation can become a skilled art piece with greater attention to the esthetic qualities of color, line, and form, even in a spontaneous art experience.

Art experiences can provide the following benefits:

☐ increase self-esteem
☐ help people of all ages to explore the future
☐ show the value of the past while reinforcing the present

- ☐ preserve personal and collective history
- ☐ aid in developing a philosophy of life
- ☐ provide a legacy for others
- ☐ help preserve a culture
- ☐ establish continuity of a human experience
- ☐ promote self-understanding
- ☐ expand consciousness
- ☐ promote self-actualization through the creative process
- ☐ explore areas of unknown potential. Instead of looking only at the individual's limitations, new areas of growth, well-being and health can be uncovered.
- ☐ help keep alive a sense of play.

The art process in itself is a private sharing between the person and the art medium.

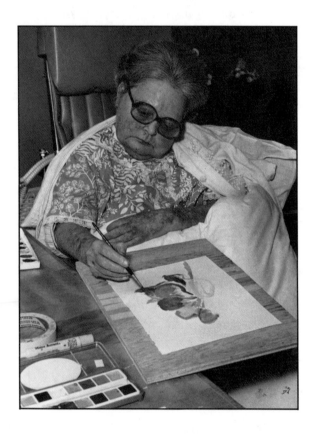

Who Can Participate

All residents. Include even a participant who physically cannot draw or write. (In this circumstance the leader may draw what participant describes, such as choice of shape, color, line and texture).

Variables which influence participants' artwork are: compatability with the group leader/therapist's ability to teach art education and study, individuals' health and ability to physically perform artwork, and participants' interest and motivation. Each of these variables can influence greatly the type and amount of activity and artwork within the creative arts session.

Size of Group

As many participants as the leader can manage sensitively. Listening to the stories told in the art medium demands individual attention. (The doodle is less personal, and we have had up to 25 people participate in this experience.)

Materials

Large sheets of blank paper; a selection of crayons, or felt-tip markers in a wide variety of colors. Make them readily available, within easy reach.

Description and Methods

Map of your own personal landscape

Leader suggests to the group: "Go back to your early childhood and make a map of your environment, your own personal landscape."

1. Imagine/visualize your front door, put a shape down in the middle of the paper (the outside of your front door, how you feel it looked). Encourage: "You're the artist, you can choose anything that represents your front door, such as an **x** or a box."
2. Color your door, the color of how you felt at that time.
3. Draw a path to your closest neighbor.
4. Draw a path or line to your school.
5. Draw another path or line to your place of worship (church, synagogue).
6. Include your secret hiding place.
7. Draw on the map the closest grocery store and the closest bus stop.
8. Now, explain your map to your partner. (Listen to the increased voice level as residents describe their early childhood landscapes!)

Notes for the Leader

In communicating with the client about his or her art experience, it is important to ask carefully worded questions which provide the "artist" with the opportunity to reveal feelings and thoughts when he or she is emotionally and psychologically ready. Like a stranger invited to a party, you ask the host, the artist, to introduce you to the art piece and show you around. The process of sharing the art experience can bring the client and health-care worker much closer as they reveal their feelings, thoughts, and concepts about their worlds and themselves.

Doodle in the sky

This exercise involves group effort, with less emphasis on the individual. Some clients may feel more secure in doodling than in doing "solo" exercises.

Ask residents to loosen their arms, the way a pitcher warms up for a baseball game, making circles. An artist needs loose muscles, no body rigidity. "Don't judge yourself, just enjoy."

Instructions:

1. Write a doodle, 2 to 3 feet in size, in the air. Choose your name, initials, or any design you like. (Take a half minute or so to think about favorite doodle.)
2. Put the doodle design in the upper right corner of a large piece of paper. Then pass the paper to the group member on the right. This person adds to the doodle and then passes the drawing to the next person. The following additions may be tried in order:

   - ☐ Expand, enlarge the doodle.
   - ☐ Fill in one area with color
   - ☐ Add texture to the doodle (inside/outside.
   - ☐ Add a happy line.
   - ☐ Add an angry line.
   - ☐ Add a joyous line. Pass.
   - ☐ Define the doodle as a picture (shape it/outline it).
   - ☐ Add other colors if suitable.
   - ☐ Finish the group doodle and give it a title.

3. Now, get some feedback. Walk around the table where the doodles are displayed. Ask how the experience felt, and do they like the picture, since no one person did the drawing.

A few suggestions:

- ☐ Keep a lively pace. Allow no more than two minutes for each phase before passing doodle to the right.

☐ Try using background music.
☐ Make available a variety of colors.
☐ Remember this is a group activity with each person contributing.

Other art activities

Crafts These include a manual skill someone would like to learn, folk art and hobbies. Examples: needlepoint, macrame, crochet, ceramics, sculpture, building or whittling with wood.

Expressive (creative) arts This involves using spontaneous art experiences in various media as a means of releasing feelings. Examples: keeping a journal or diary using drawings (or writings) to express and keep track of feelings and thoughts such as daily joys, troubles, gifts, pains. This journal can help point out the meaning and value in one's everyday life. Suggestion: Tack a large piece of paper to the resident's bedroom wall to write or draw images, feelings and thoughts. Ask visitors or staff also to write and draw on the paper, sharing their thoughts and feelings.

Skill learning in art This means learning how to draw, paint, sculpt, or use other techniques with various media as an art form. It also involves learning how to see the esthetic qualities of design, color, form, and beauty of nature. Examples: painting with watercolors, acrylics, oils; drawing with pastels, craypas, crayons, colored pencils, inks; sculpting with clay, making projects in plaster of Paris; doing collages and murals, and learning other art skills. Studying the work of other artists and art styles can broaden one's horizon of ideas and knowledge about art and life.

Notes for the Leader

Upon finishing an art product, the artist/client should be invited to discuss and disclose his or her feelings about the art activity, the art product, or feelings which arose during the creative experience. Remember, art activity (creative process) in itself can be very therapeutic; the product is not the only reward.

While the work is in progress, try to resist offering help unless it's requested. The art experience should be a reflection of the artist as much as possible, with little assistance from others whose influence may interfere with the creative process of self-expression.

Using art with adults in a relaxed, non-judgmental and non-threatening manner can help people share their feelings and thoughts, nonverbally on paper and verbally in discussion. Feelings and thoughts which may be difficult to express in words can be unlocked through art. The art process in itself is a private sharing between the person and the art medium. In this experience each individual has the opportunity to be unique without concern about being questioned, evaluated, criticized or rejected. The art medium always accepts the "artist" unconditionally, waiting to be molded and shaped to the individual's liking. Hence, the resident becomes master of his or her universe, the creative process and product.

If you find resistance to art, remember that many residents were raised in a setting where free creative expression was not encouraged and perhaps even actively discouraged. Try to break through these barriers by leading a discussion on expression. What were the conventional attitudes when residents were growing up? Did they ever experience creative, flowing expression? How did it feel?

Other important suggestions for health-care professionals who conduct art experiences:

- ☐ Have good art materials available and make sure the participant becomes familiar with them.
- ☐ Find out what the participant's expectations may be and what the activity is designed for.
- ☐ Offer encouragement, but don't be pushy or overhelpful. Know when to be quiet.
- ☐ Be prepared to offer different art activities if the one you had in mind doesn't suit the participant.
- ☐ Don't make the activity seem childish. It can be fun, but always treat the participant as an adult.
- ☐ Become familiar with the art materials and get some exposure to art experience. The staff person does not have to be an expert—you and the participant can learn together.
- ☐ Develop spontaneity on your own. You are the tool to help the participant express his creativity.
- ☐ Don't do the same activity every day, but do use a range of art experiences. Do not, however, go on to another activity before you have completed the one you are working on, unless you have a good reason to change activities.
- ☐ Be prepared to give a meaningful introduction to the session, to help with creating art during the middle of the session, and convey a sense of finishing at the end of the session with discussion and possible future plans.

□ Be prepared to discuss esthetics, the value of art, and the value of looking at things in new ways.
□ Introduce discussion about art and life. These discussions don't have to be a critique of participants' art work if that is too threatening.
□ Develop a sense of process, continuity, commitment, and love in the art process and in your relationship with the participant.
□ Recognize and accept those who need to produce a pretty product. If the client wants to feel he or she has made something useful, help to achieve this goal.

Remember, any and every art expression is valid and meaningful. We are concerned with wellness, review of life, a way of understanding and practicing creativity in old age. No matter how creativity is expressed, *everyone wins*.

Ribbon/Circle Game

Purpose

The objective of this game is literally to unite the members of the group, with each person holding on to a long ribbon that is formed into a circle.

Who Can Participate

Every resident should participate in this activity. Those who are able to stand should do so, and those unable to stand can participate in a chair within the circle. Because the ribbon is soft and stretches readily, even those with arthritis or pain from other sources can still be part of the game.

Size of Group

There is no limit to the group size, since the ribbon can be extended as necessary.

The ribbon/circle game can help to strengthen the sense of community among group members.

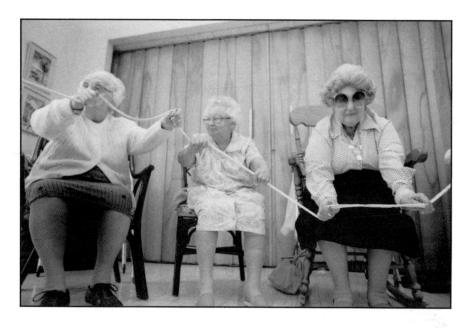

Materials

The ribbon is made up of several Ace (elastic) bandages sewn together. The ultimate length of the ribbon depends on the group size. This elastic material is particularly suitable for this purpose, since it stretches in all directions and does not break or tear because of various stresses.

Description and Methods

The residents are asked to stand or be seated in a large circle. The ribbon is then threaded around the circle. Every member is asked to hold on to the ribbon so that it unites the group. It is sometimes helpful to suggest that the energy of the entire group flows through the ribbon, and even those who have little energy will feel the benefit of the union. The ribbon/circle game can be combined with music, which encourages reaching and stretching while holding on to the ribbon.

Play and Laughter

Life does not cease to be funny when people die, neither does it cease to be serious when people laugh.

Purpose

Therapeutic benefits have been attributed to the use of laughter and humor in combatting stress and in supporting rehabilitation from illness. Dr. Robert Butler, head of the Department of Geriatrics at Mt. Sinai Hospital in New York, cites humor as an adaptive technique and applauds the work of Norman Cousins, author of *The Anatomy of an Illness*. Cousins, writing about the healing power of humor and laughter, reviews the physiological effects of negative emotions such as fear, rage, and frustration. He observes that blood vessels constrict and there is often an excess flow of hydrochloric acid in the stomach with these emotional states. On the other hand, laughter, joy, and similar positive emotions produce greater blood flow, muscular relaxation, and a sense of relief from stress. Positive emotions may therefore be considered as helpful tools in promoting health.

We know how laughter and humor affect our personal lives. They help us to lighten our day, build relationships, and feel good about ourselves. Humor also helps encourge creativity. Developing an attitude not of "grin and bear it" but "grin and share it" improves communication and problem solving. Phrases such as "humor can add light years to your life"; "remember, laughing matters"; "how's your laugh life?" and "laughter is the shortest distance between two people" are easily applicable in the lives of the elderly. Yet all too often humor seems to be in short supply, especially in the lives of the five percent of the population who are in nursing homes. Laughter, play, and comedy are desperately needed in this setting.

We define play as any activity that tends to produce the emotion of joy or the experience of "having fun." Play and humor can be injected into group activity throughout the session, not just when focusing on humor as an issue.

Who Can Participate

In a group setting, residents will respond to laughter. The enjoyment and sharing of humor help build group solidarity and can encourage the reluctant participant to relax.

101

Materials	**Audiotapes**

"Just for Laughs" (45 minutes of continuous laughter, recorded live)
"Funny Business" – PO Box 3000-333A, Santa Barbara, California 93130
"Anatomy of an Illness - The Healing Power of Humor" - Norman
    Cousins, 4370 Alpine Rd., Partola Valley, California 94025

Other Materials

"Laughing Matters," (magazine) Humor Project – Sagamore Institute,
    110 Spring Street, Saratoga Springs, New York 12866
Balloons - Edmund Scientific Co., 101 E. Gloucester Pike,
    Barrington, New Jersey 09007

**Description
and Methods**

Laughter Tape

Encourage group laughing and tape it on an audio recorder. When
you play it back, have another recorder ready to catch the laughter
as the group hears their own laughter. Laughter is infectious. There
are several laughter tapes (see above) that can be used to induce
laughter. After the group listens to the laughter, ask for feedback at
once: "How do you feel?" "Do your feel heavier?" "Do you feel
lighter?" "Did you think of pain?" "Did you forget your pain?"

Include laughter in as many activities as possible, even if you as
staff must laugh at yourself. Be a clown! Being vulnerable to being
laughed *at* usually evokes being laughed *with*.

Try This

Have a discussion about laughter and play as methods essential to
health. Ask what laughter does (guide residents to answers like:
relaxes the body, reduces pain, stimulates the body, mind and spirit,
puts new perspectives on problems). Talk about how negative
thoughts, beliefs and emotions can be depressive and how our
positive thoughts can promote healing. Explain how laughter and
play are among the first things that go when a person is ill, at a
time when it is most needed.

Try This

Ask for a list of things that produce laughter and are playful—you can collect and read them, or better yet, have each person express their own joys, things they enjoy doing now or have enjoyed in the past. You may get answers such as comedy acts, the circus, the Marx brothes, Jack Benny, cards, games, telling jokes. Encourage each person to tell a funny story. Keep stressing that play was essential in the past and is no less essential now.

Try This

Balloons are always fun to play with. Ask the residents to try to balance balloons on their heads, or to juggle the balloons.

Ask for the funniest situation, biggest laugh, funniest movie the residents have seen to set the stage before you use the laughter tape with the group.

Laughter is the shortest distance between two people.

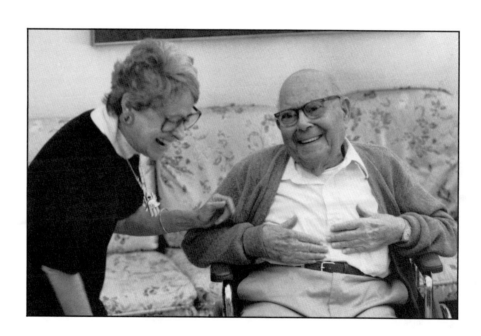

Notes for the Leader

You may want to discuss negative connotations about play with the group! We were taught early in life to stop playing. Parents said, "You're playing too much, you're lazy, you could make better use of your time, you're wasting time." Mature people understand the importance of play and ignore the old adage that play is sinful, that work is good but play is bad.

True play is wonderful pleasure. Many of us deny ourselves pleasure—we don't do enough things that truly bring us joy. We often tell ourselves that play can wait. "I must get the job finished,"; "Playing is for kids," "That is just being silly" are common refrains. We tend to play and laugh less and less, particularly when illness occurs; this is truly unfortunate because illness is a time when laughing really matters. "You don't stop playing when you grow old—you grow old when you stop playing."

Remember, laughing is not only contagious, but powerful. Shared laughter can create bonds between people and break through the barriers of isolation.

Parachute Play

Purpose

By standing or sitting in a circle with a large open parachute, the residents unite as a group and experience the pleasure of being together. In addition, the raising and lowering of the parachute provides gentle and invigorating exercise and encourages deep breathing. Each of the participants can make a contribution to the group effort, with visible results.

Who Can Participate

All residents are able to stand or sit holding a parachute; no one has to be excluded.

Size of Group

The size of the group depends on the size of parachute. If the number of residents exceeds the available space, simply divide the group into smaller sections, with each taking a turn.

Materials

A used or surplus parachute can be obtained in most Army/Navy stores or surplus outlets. The parachutes come in many sizes—the larger the parachute, the better.

Description and Methods

Ask residents to sit or stand in a circle around the parachute, with everyone holding on to its edges. At the leader's cue, the participants take a deep breath as they swoop the parachute up into the air, making it billow like a sail. Then, as they exhale, everyone drops their arms—still holding on—allowing the parachute to collapse gently to the floor. Repeat the cycle several times, or until participants tire.

Provide the residents with balloons, which they throw towards the center of the parachute before raising it in the air. The object is to try to get the balloons through the center hole at the top of the parachute.

One-To-One Visits

Purpose

The leader should visit each resident individually at fairly regular intervals. These visits are an excellent means to reach residents, reinforce new learning and help motivate each person to participate in group programs. In addition, visiting helps the leader identify the needs of individuals that may not be clearly understood in a group setting. Also, it is an excellent time to allow residents to express their feelings about life changes they have experienced with institutional living.

Who Can Participate

Residents at every level should be visited. The leader should allocate sufficient time for visiting, always starting with new residents with whom an early visit is mandatory.

Materials

None.

Description and Methods

☐ A visit is an opportunity to start building a trust relationship with a new resident. Be sure to keep any commitments you make, in order to preserve this trust.

☐ During your visit, arrange seating so that you are face-to-face with the resident, allowing good eye contact. If the resident permits it, you can make some physical contact as well—a touch on the hand or shoulder, for example.

☐ Always listen for the language of wellness. Even with new residents who are suffering from loss, fear, anxiety or anger, there are words that tell of times when things went well. These are valuable clues. For example, "I liked to read, but I can't go to the library any more." Here, the leader should pursue the resident's lead by finding out what kind of books she enjoys and arranging to obtain the books. (Does the resident have vision problems? Get large-print books or books on tape and arrange for the use of a tape player.)

☐ Make a specific plan for the resident to perform exercises in bed or in the chair. Otherwise the exercise program may never be implemented.

☐ Introduce the resident to other members of the group or to nursing home personnel, encouraging new friendships.

☐ Identify support systems that the resident may need and try to have a social worker, volunteers, or even other residents perform these roles.

☐ A visit is a good time to give the new resident a plant and ask her to water and nurture it every day. The plant represents life and growth.

Notes for the Leader

Regardless of what else may be accomplished during a one-on-one visit, the following guidelines are important:

☐ Encourage self-responsibility and self-care.

☐ Help new residents express their feelings about the changes they have experienced in their lives. Find out specifically what has changed; what losses they feel most.

☐ Remember, the new resident may not speak openly at the first visit, but continued interaction will bring trust.

☐ Try to meet with family members and include them in the group. Many family members enjoy such participation and learn skills that help them cope.

This resident had been depressed. Careful listening during the first one-to-one visit helped the leader to reframe the resident's concerns into positive goals. (Note good eye contact, which is essential for one-to-one visits.)

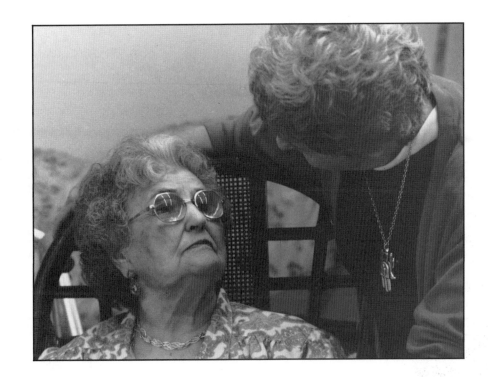

Other Issues

Confusion

Confusion resulting from emotional or physical causes is a frequent and almost common occurrence among elderly people living in nursing homes, hospitals and long-term care facilities. Confusion or disorientation can be defined as an impairment of orientation (time, person, place), usually in conjunction with one or more of the following symptoms: impairment of memory of recent and/or past events; impairment of comprehension, judgment and self-expression; emotional lability (overactivity and easy arousal to tears or laughter); and distortion of perceived reality and awareness of self. The term "confusion" is often used as a catch-all label to signify symptoms that may be due to organic illnesses or to a combination of social, psychological and physical conditions. Put differently, disorientation in the elderly may well be the result of arteriosclerosis (organic brain syndrome), Alzheimer's disease, or other organic mental disorder, but it may also be due to psychosocial factors on their own. Indeed, it is often hard to determine how much of a person's confusion is related to organic disease and how much to social and psychological causes.

Another factor that contributes to disorientation is labeling. Once an elderly person is described or classified as confused or mentally disabled, there is a tendency for him to act out the part, fulfilling the expectations of others while negating or giving up ego strength. Adding to this problem is that older people receive much more personal attention when they show signs of illness, helplessness or disorientation. This attention-getting mechanism may indirectly contribute to the state of confusion.

Those responsible for the care of patients with confusion must delineate the origin of the problem in order to manage it successfully. Is the disorientation due to organic or psychosocial causes? This allows the care giver to focus on the reversible aspects of each.

Confusion Related to Loss and Life Changes

As a person ages, his life changes in many ways, and he may encounter more losses than gains at a certain stage. Among the losses are: loss of job (retirement); loss of spouse (or of spouse's mental and physical ability); loss of home; loss of financial security; and loss of one's physical and mental capacities. These losses cover a wide spectrum of social, psychological and physical conditions and are difficult to handle individually, let alone collectively. It is not uncommon for people who are unable to make a positive transition through these life changes to become depressed. Confusion in the elderly is often a manifestation of depression, which is usually amenable to treatment. After the depression lifts, greater clarity of expression and more normal behavior may be observed. The point is that the social and psychological losses that accompany aging can lead to or exaggerate confusion, and that this state is reversible.

Confusion and Longevity Therapy

How does the Longevity Therapy program deal with confused people? This question arises repeatedly, since confusion is certainly one of the most common problems in nursing homes. Indeed, in many facilities as many as 50% of the residents may be confused at some time or other. Should all of these patients be excluded from the program?

We do not automatically exclude from our sessions anyone who is confused. This would be a sad mistake because, not infrequently, some residents whose confusion results from psychosocial causes or depression show signs of improvement during Longevity Therapy. The very nature of the program serves to mitigate adverse social and psychological factors that contribute to confusion. If a resident is mildly confused, we specifically ask him if he would like to participate in the program. On the other hand, if the resident is grossly confused and disruptive to the program, no attempt is made to enlist him. In reaching a decision about the participation of confused people, it is important to consider the attitude of the group leader. If the leader feels uncomfortable in dealing with confused residents, it is probably wiser to focus instead on alert, mentally clear individuals. On the other hand, the group leader should make an effort to include at least mildly confused residents as much as possible, recognizing that their successful participation can be beneficial not only for themselves, but for the entire group, including the leader.

Death and Dying

It is unrealistic to discuss nursing homes and not to consider the process of dying and the reality of death. Despite the tremendous contribution of Dr. Elisabeth Kübler-Ross and others to our understanding of the dying process, many of us have great difficulty facing the death of other people and the idea of our own eventual death.

Our denial of death has a profound impact on the terminally ill patient and will have a profound impact on our relationship to the residents of the nursing home. For many residents, nursing homes are the end stage of life. Our own fears of death make it difficult for us to help these elders through this last stage of life and through the dying process. When we accept and can openly talk about death and dying, the residents will not feel that they have to hide from their inevitable end. Death is a natural process of living.

Dr. Kübler-Ross utilized a simple technique to allow a terminally ill patient to communicate. She asks the simple question, "How long did you know?" We in nursing homes can use this question also, and we can ask "Do you think about death? Do you think about your own dying? What do you want for yourself?" As part of our work we see residents pass through various stages of health and into the final stage of life. Indeed, nursing home staff often become the family for a terminally ill person.

There are two important tasks for the nursing home staff to undertake during the stage of dying: First, to make the person comfortable, and second, to make the person feel loved and cared for. Kübler-Ross emphasizes that controlling the pain of an ill person is of primary importance. The physical need of pain control must be met by round-the-clock medication, preferably oral medication. Nearly all physicians agree that the goal is to keep the person not only comfortable, but alert. With the effective use of drugs the terminally ill person can be aware and be a part of the dying process. The idea is not to overmedicate and obtund the patient but to keep pain under control, and allow the person to remain in control of his/her thoughts during the final stages of life.

During this period the patient needs to be listened to, to be touched, and to be given unconditional love. Kübler-Ross suggests that a hospitalized patient should go home to die; those who have lived in a nursing home, however, may feel that they are already home. Wherever the person is, the family and nursing staff should encourage any form of communication, spoken or symbolic. Listening with the heart to the dying in order to help them complete their unfinished business and unexpressed wishes, holding them, and touching them are all that is needed. Being present for the terminally ill, silently touching, helping them express themselves, and interpreting their wishes should be our role.

None of these thoughts is especially new or profound, it is just that we sometimes forget them. It is natural to help the dying person depart from life with a feeling of being cared for and loved. Much like a newborn who is held, rocked, and given unconditional love, so should the dying be given the same loving consideration. Life's entrance and exit have much the same meaning—a new transition—and much the same need: loving care. The dying need to be listened to with the heart.

Section Three

Group Work
with Elders

Group Work

As explained in Section One of this book, Longevity Therapy is based on group activity. The benefits of a group have been described under "Group Building." The object of this chapter is to consider some practical issues involved in forming a group and in implementing group activity.

Before proceeding, let us review some fundamental approaches to working with elders (in contrast to younger age groups). Special factors to be considered include:

- ☐ Leaders must use a more directive approach in dealing with the elderly in group programs. The roles of group members in each activity should be explained carefully.
- ☐ Physical problems, including motor and sensory losses, must be taken into account in determining what a resident can and cannot do in group programs.
- ☐ Leaders must provide far more support, encourgement and empathy than they might provide in working with younger people.
- ☐ Leaders should function as an integral part of the group and share themselves with the members.
- ☐ Recognizing that the composition of the groups may vary from session to session (because of indisposition or illness of certain residents), efforts must be made to preserve contact with the remaining members of the group during the absence of their friends.

Starting a Group

Before contacting potentially suitable members for a group, the following decisions must be made:

- ☐ Who will be the leader and co-leader of the group?
- ☐ The time and place of each session
- ☐ Duration of sessions
- ☐ How long a group will continue to function
- ☐ The purposes of particular groups
- ☐ Staff support required to carry out activities.

Choosing Potential Members

In selecting particular residents to be part of a group, it is essential that the person himself wants to be part of the group, not that the leader wants him to be. Also, a resident who is likely to disrupt a group because of behavioral problems should not be included in an otherwise sound group.

Other factors to consider in selecting group members are:

- [ ] medical diagnosis
- [ ] functional capacity
- [ ] physical status
- [ ] communication skills
- [ ] general affect
- [ ] mobility.

Session Planning

Prior to each session the leader and co-leader should discuss the intention and purpose of the day's activity. Most sessions require some materials or props to conduct the activity, and these must be assembled and set up in advance of the session.

Most of the activities described in this book require at least two leaders. The group leader directs the activity while the co-leader, in addition to helping, also analyzes the group process and solves problems and conflicts that arise. The skills required of the leader and co-leader are described in the next section.

Response to Program

The leader and co-leader should make a deliberate effort to evaluate each resident before and during the series of group activities.

Especially important is to assess changes in mood, alertness, memory, and orientation of each individual. Remember that modification of behavior may be slight or slow, but may be occurring nevertheless. Periodically, the leaders should compare their conclusions about the progress of each resident with the opinions of the general staff, who have an opportunity to observe the residents in a different light.

Check List For Group Planning

1. Decide on the *Group Focus* for the day. This theme defines the activities for the day and helps clarify the leader's goals.

2. Start the day's program with *Check-In*. The feedback the residents provide at the beginning of the session allows the leader to determine individual moods and needs. Be flexible and build on the material generated by the group members, even though it may be different from the group focus for the day. Rigidity in planning can be defeating.

3. Adhere to the basic tenets of the Longevity Therapy Program, regardless of the activity being performed:

☐ **Encouragement** Discouragement is a major disease in nursing homes, and every effort should be made to encourage the residents. The encouragement must be sincere and appropriate.

☐ **Responsibility** The importance of being responsible and making decisions should be stressed at every opportunity. Indeed, the need and the right to be responsible is one of the uppermost themes of Longevity Therapy.

☐ **Responsible Dependency** Elders should be independent as long as possible, but then learn to accept needed assistance graciously from others.

☐ **Self-Awareness** The uniqueness of each individual must be identified and then encouraged. A group is a good setting to foster self-awareness.

☐ **Expression** Among the highest priorities of the program is to encourage residents to express their feelings. Pent-up, unspoken emotions cause tension. Once these are expressed, the body and mind are freer.

☐ **Community Spirit** We exist and survive by sharing and caring for each other. A strong community spirit is fundamental to all activities.

4. Observe carefully. Keep your eyes and ears open for changes in the residents' ways and attitudes. Even minor changes may be meaningful.

5. Use positive language. The manner in which the leader acts and speaks to the group and to individuals is a powerful force in the success of the program. Try to be open, friendly, inviting, enthusiastic, supportive and non-judgmental in dealing with residents. A smiling approach is wonderful medicine.

6. Encourage feedback. This important interaction between leader and participant allows each to become aware of the needs and preferences of the other.

7. Suggest homework. Always encourage the elder's capacity to be active and try new things. Suggest practicing the activities they enjoy after the group session.

8. Encourage movement and physical activity. Remember, movement helps physical disabilities, improves muscle tone, stimulates energy, benefits the heart, and brings the body and mind into harmony.

9. Adopt a sound belief system about caring for the elderly. The system should reflect your philosophy concerning optimal care in a nursing home environment. Some typical elements of an effective belief system include:

☐ "Growth can occur at 80 as well as 8." (Flexibility and growth must continue throughout life to combat the changes and losses accompanying aging.)

☐ New information can be learned at any age, even past 80 or 90 years.

☐ Aging is a developmental stage of living, a time to review and accept one's life, not a time to hide or retreat.

☐ Growing old should be an active process. Each person has an obligation to act on his or her own behalf in order to function with fewer support systems (family members, friends) and diminished health.

10. Dignify and honor the elderly for the wisdom they have accumulated over their long lives.

Representative Group Activities

On the following pages are suggestions for group sessions, each organized around a central theme. You can adapt them to suit the requirements of your group. Note that each session is designed to include all the components discussed in Part 1: Philosophy, Movement, Expression, Feedback, Motivation, and Group Building.

Use these examples as starting points for planning your own group sessions. Remember, what happens in one session can be a factor in planning the next one. Each group is a unique constellation of individuals, and the dynamics of groups will vary accordingly.

Group Focus:
Early Morning Exercises in Bed

Check-In

"What did you do the first thing this morning while still in bed?"

Discussion

Key point: Start the day in a positive way with early morning exercises, while still in bed. Not only will the exercises increase your muscle tone, but they provide pleasure by allowing you to move and function with greater ease. Deciding to start the day by exercising involves making a choice. Choices are important, since it is only by making sound, positive choices that we can enjoy life and free ourselves of pain and tension.

Activities

Demonstrate physical exercises that the residents can perform in bed by themselves (*see* Exercises in Bed). The extent of the exercises must be tailored to the residents' health and physical ability.

Stretch exercises in conjunction with breathing exercises should be modelled by the leader.

The exercises are more fun when performed with upbeat jazz music.

Ending

Continue to play music and allow residents to express themselves in body movement.

Homework

Remember that movement can be as little as moving your fingers or as much as walking down to the dining room to be with others. Keep moving!

Group Focus:
Touch

Check-In

Ask everyone to assume a good posture and breathe deeply (*see* Section Two, Body Image). Name something you touched today that you care about.

Discussion

Talk about touch. Suggest that everyone massage his/her roommate's hand. Try to break barriers and listen to problems and complaints of others. Discuss difficulties we have in touching and trusting each other.

Activities

☐ *Love tapping* Partners lightly tap their neighbor's hand and shoulders.
☐ *Yoga* Focus on hand exercises.
☐ *Movement* Ribbon movements with music; ribbon game.
☐ *Massage* Pair up and massage each other's hands.

Ending

Group singing. Ask for requests; let group make as many choices as possible.

Group Focus:
Music and Emotions

Check-In

Ask each resident about his favorite music.

Discussion

Play music of different types with varying tempos and moods, while the group listens. After each segment, ask the residents how the music makes them feel (sad, happy, angry, sleepy, energetic). As you know, people have many different tastes, so do respect the individuality of responses.

Activities

Move to Music

Select a medley of your choice; include peppy music, sad music and so forth. While listening, the leader should move along with the residents in response to the different sounds and tempos. For residents who are chairbound or not fully mobile, movement of the arms and hands can serve the purpose.

Music and Poetry

Create a group poem from the residents' verbal responses to the music they hear (*see* Section Two, Music). Remember that the poem is meant to be no more than an expression of emotions and thoughts; little else matters. After the poem is written and read to the group, discuss with the residents what the process of expressing the music as word images was like. Encourage the group by acknowledging how fine a poem they created.

Ending

Close the session with ribbon movements accompanied by music (we often select "Some of These Days" as the music for this activity). Ask the group to "stretch," "swing," "reach in and out" with a long ribbon (*see* Section Two, Ribbon/Circle game).

Homework

Listen to the radio. Which sounds do you like most? Does your choice differ at different times of the day? Consider what effect music has on you. Share your thoughts with the group at the next session.

Case History

A depressed, newly-admitted patient was invited to participate in a Longevity Therapy group. She declined to do so, and we respected her right to refuse. One day we brought live jazz to the nursing home, and I watched her express her enjoyment by keeping rhythm with the music. The music was such a motivator for her that when I asked her to dance with me, she accepted immediately. She didn't stop dancing that day! The music allowed her to feel comfortable with new people, and shortly she joined in the other groups. She started to take a leadership role, helping those less able than she. Music was the motivator.

Group Focus:
Self-Healing and Visualization

Check-In

"What is your healing color? Red? Blue? White?"

Discussion

As explained in Section Two, Visualization is an excellent method for relaxation and meditation. Here, we are attempting to use color and guided imagery to help healing, using a white light as a healing force.

Activities

Play

Make up a simple game with your own rules so everyone wins. For example, try using a parachute and a Nerf ball: let participants put their heads in the center of the parachute and take turns ducking the Nerf ball. Make up consequences. Have fun! Remind the group that when a person is having fun, nothing hurts. Play allows release of tension and helps us feel good!

Imagery

Suggestion Sit relaxed, but not rigid, with the spine straight enough for an imaginary white beam of light to pass through each vertebra, as if grounding you to the earth and attaching you to a star. Imagine that this white light has healing properties. When you inhale, imagine this white light passing through your body to each area, to the ankles, the feet, the toes. Imagine the white light surrounding your calf, knee, thigh, surrounding the torso, the fingers, hands, arms, shoulders, neck, face and head. With each breath let the white light fill your entire being, healing and cleansing you. Concentrate on the light and remember its healing power.

Ending

Lead group in the song, "Somewhere Over the Rainbow."

Homework

Think about the white light and, tonight, allow yourself to experience it again.

Group Focus:
Winning

Check-In	"What would make you feel especially good today?"
Discussion	A winning situation is one in which you accomplish something that makes you feel healthier and happier, and makes you like yourself. Winning has many facets. Taking responsibility for yourself, for example, is winning. By doing activities such as morning bed exercises, breathing exercises, being aware of your posture, you are taking responsibility; this is winning. Another example of winning is to bring your feelings out in the open—not hide them—and to express yourself. You can be much happier with a winning attitude.
Activities	(*see* Section Two for fuller description)
	☐ Breathing Exercises ☐ Love Tapping ☐ Echo Game ☐ Emotional Chorus (*see* Encouraging Emotional Expression)
Ending	Music that brightens the spirit.
Case History	Mrs. P. a 90-year-young resident of a nursing home, had serious high blood pressure. Through participation in Longevity Therapy sessions, she learned to reduce her blood pressure by practicing deep yoga breathing and thereby avoided hospitalization. This success is a "win."

Group Focus:
Hands

Check-In	Name one thing your hands did for you today.
Discussion	Hands are for helping. Ask "What gift you could give yourelf today?" Pair off. Listen to each other's answers.
Activities	☐ Move hands to music "Raindrops Are Falling." ☐ Give everyone an imaginary baton and let them conduct the music, using arms, hands, fingers. ☐ Yoga hand exercises (*see* Section Two, Yoga). ☐ Ask residents to pair off and exchange hand massages.
Ending	Lead group in song "Listen, Listen."
Homework	Do one thing for yourself today. Suggestion: massage hands; sing in shower; relaxation and breathing exercises; make a friend of a new resident.

Group Focus:
Sharing Feelings

Check-In

Ask each resident to tell what emotion is uppermost in his/her feelings today. Happiness? Sadness? Anger? (The leader should write down the responses and deal with them individually during the session.)

Discussion

The underlying idea of this session is to make it clear that all of us must have someone to share our thoughts. The key is friendship. Acknowledge that it is often difficult to express our true feelings to another person, but the rewards are worth it. Try to find one member of the group and talk to him/her about yourself.

Activities

☐ *"Ha" Breath* With exhalation and intent you can throw out negative emotions. See if it works for you.

☐ *Making Faces* Exaggerate some common emotions using facial expressions: for instance, "clown up" the emotions of a sad person and an angry person. Make certain that the group understands that you are *not* making fun of anyone in the group or belittling the emotional reality of a situation. Making faces may help a person laugh at himself and perhaps gain some perspective about his emotional feelings.

☐ *Music* The song "Can't We Be Friends" by Ella Fitzgerald and Louis Armstrong is a good choice for this group focus. Stretching movements can be included with the music.

Ending

Song: "From You I Receive, To You I Give."

Group Focus:
Play

Check-In

"What are your favorite games?"

Discussion

Play does many good things for you. It makes you feel brighter, forget your worries, and lightens your load. It also helps relieve pain and stress, and many believe it promotes healing. Think about it: Play is a pretty easy way to feel better in a hurry!

Activities

- [ ] *Clowning with Balloons* Balance large balloons on the heads of the participants. Throw a balloon to each person in the group and ask, "What kind of humor makes you laugh?" (Jokes, other laughter, slapstick, movies, comedians?) Note each person's reactions.
- [ ] Play a laughter tape (*see* Section Two, Play and Laughter).
- [ ] *Art* Try doodling and let the group see the results (*see* Section Two, Art).
- [ ] *Parachute Play* Use parachute for therapeutic and joyous range-of-motion exercise.

Ending

Song: "From You I Receive/To You I Give/Together We Share/and From This We Live."

Homework

Ask the residents to think of a playful story to tell the group during the next visit.

Group Focus:
Laughter

Check-In   "What tree do you feel like today? What flower? What color?"

Discussion   Ask what laughter does: How do you feel after you laugh? Does any area of your body feel tight after you laugh? Explain how laughter contributes to wellness.

Activities

☐ *Laughter tape*   Playing a laughter tape sets the tone and relaxes everyone.

☐ *Feedback*   What did you notice when you laughed? Did you become relaxed?

☐ *Movement*   Gentle stretching and breathing which focuses on tight areas of body (as described by participants).

☐ *Reminiscence*   Pair off as partners and prime the memory bank with funny stories of your life.

Ending   Play or sing a light song. Ask for suggestions.

Group Focus:
Self-responsibility

Check-In	Echo Game (*see* Section Two, Check-In).
Discussion	Consider different ways to assume self-responsibility. Remember, it's everybody's right to be responsible! (Self-care, grooming, being active, are all forms of self-responsibility.)
Activities	☐ *Music:* "Down by the Riverside." Move to words; ask participants to stretch, shake, and bend. ☐ Keep group united with a long ribbon (*see* Section Two, Ribbon/Circle Game). Suggest we also can help others and assume responsibility in this way.
Ending	Have each participant offer one way they will be self-responsible this week.

Section Four

Training

Group Leaders and Their Training

Clearly, the effectiveness of the Longevity Therapy program depends for the most part on the ability and enthusiasm of the group leader. Unless the group leader has the energy, sensitivity and know-how to bring out the inherent capabilities of the residents, the program can have little meaning.

The group activities comprising Longevity Therapy demand active, motivated leaders. All leaders must possess certain traits and skills, many of which may be already in place, and others which must be learned by appropriate training. Here are some of the characteristics we believe are important for those who have chosen, or who want to be, a Longevity Therapy group leader:

Qualities of a Group Leader

- ☐ Is friendly, even-tempered, warm, and above all, shows a high degree of compassion and sensitivity to others
- ☐ Can organize and manage several tasks at once without being overwhelmed
- ☐ Works with a sense of kindness and empathy toward elders, not pity
- ☐ Has the patience necessary to help elders help themselves, rather than do the task in their behalf
- ☐ Exerts creativity, resourcefulness and initiative
- ☐ Seeks potential and possibilities for improvement at all times in dealing with elders
- ☐ Perseveres and holds to beliefs, even in the face of obstacles
- ☐ Recognizes that change often occurs slowly and gradually and is willing to wait out results
- ☐ Takes responsibility for own actions and does not project blame on others
- ☐ Appreciates the value of every individual's response, negative or positive, and uses that response to uncover underlying meanings
- ☐ Shows tactfulness in dealing with others, even though this may be difficult to accomplish

☐ Accepts directives and criticisms
☐ Functions effectively outside rigidly structured settings and demonstrates flexibility when necessary
☐ Shows enthusiasm and expressiveness with even small triumphs
☐ Recognizes that helping others make changes is not only an enjoyable endeavor, but that it serves the recipient well
☐ Conducts his or her own personal program of care relative to diet, exercise, and achieving a spirit of wellness.

Becoming a Group Leader

In most programs group leaders are selected from the staff of the institution. Particularly suitable for the role of group leaders are staff members in social work, nursing, occupational therapy, art and music therapy, and recreational therapy. All of these disciplines provide excellent training in their own right and would serve well for the education of group leaders. However, other staff members can be trained as group leaders, particularly if they have many of the characteristics mentioned above and are highly motivated and enthusiastic about their work.

For those who wish to develop a self-educational plan to function as group leaders, the following guidelines are helpful, in our experience:

☐ Clarify your own beliefs, ideals and goals; decide whether you have the motivation to learn and serve as a group leader.
☐ Observe groups in action and try to develop your own skills in expression, play, art, music and movement.
☐ Learn to speak and present material in a group setting. Small lectures, discussion groups and demonstrations are good ways to start.
☐ Observe people very carefully, including their body language, and learn to recognize even the smallest changes in behavior. This is a particularly important skill, since detecting behavioral changes often determines whether the program is effective for a particular person.
☐ Learn to describe what you see and hear; this feedback may be of great value to the other members of the team and is of prime importance.
☐ Learn to assess the capabilities of the group members so that activities can be planned accordingly.
☐ Learn how to involve each resident in the group activity; remember that each person is unique and that different

approaches are necessary for different people.

☐ Spend time with individuals who have difficulty in expressing themselves clearly and learn to communicate with them.

☐ Try to learn about the normal aging process and about the way illness affects elders. Always remember that unusual behavioral patterns may be due to illness and medications and are not necessarily related to old age itself.

The Team Approach to Group Leadership

In identifying personnel to serve as group leaders, it is important to realize that existing members of the professional staff may already have excellent skills on which to base a training program in Longevity Therapy. In most institutions there is a good chance of finding a nurse or a social worker or an allied health professional who has a reasonably good understanding of fundamental concepts of dealing with the elderly, such as psychological aspects of aging, group dynamics, verbal and nonverbal forms of expression, or experience with organized physical activity and movement.

We have found it beneficial to organize a team of staff members, each of whom may have a different talent or ability, so that the members of the team stimulate and train each other in their particular disciplines. In other words, one staff member may have useful knowledge about the psychological aspects of aging, while a second member is trained in occupational therapy, and a third member is experienced in art and music. By sharing their collective knowledge, the members train each other so that well-rounded group leaders may emerge. The concepts and methods of Longevity Therapy described in this book can readily serve as the basis of a broad training program. (A bibliography to help locate additional training resources is found at the end of the book.)

This in-house program should be supplemented by organized group instruction. For example, if one person on the team is knowledgeable about Yoga exercises, she or he should conduct classes in Yoga for the others. In the event no one is experienced in a particular field, the team can locate a Yoga teacher, for instance, in the community to provide instruction to the group. (Some suggestions for utilizing community resources to provide appropriate teachers are discussed below.) Although this piecemeal approach to in-house training may seem much less than ideal, the results are surprisingly good, and many excellent group leaders have received their training in this manner. Fundamental to this premise is the need to function as a team and for other members of the nursing home staff to be included in the overall effort. By involving all members of the staff in the team's goals and purposes, the program achieves greater acceptance and encouragement. Indeed, it is a good practice to invite all nursing home staff members to various group activities so that they can understand the benefits to the residents and the personal rewards that come with this type of participation. Group leaders and other staff members should, as suggested through this book, "try on" each experience—whether it be Yoga or breathing exercises—for themselves. The results often become a strong motivational force.

Supplemental Training

It is evident that the self-training program described above is only a starting point and serves primarily as a base to build knowledge. In large institutions the diversity of the staff may be sufficient to allow a training program to be carried out from within, with staff members in different fields training each other. More often, however, other resources are needed, especially in smaller institutions, where the availability of personnel is limited. In the latter situation, several supplemental means, especially community resources, may be used. These include:

☐ Teachers of Yoga, Tai Chi and New Games can often be located through YMCAs, continuing adult education programs, health centers, recreation departments, and similar sources. Artists, musicians, poets and mimes within the community are often willing to come to a nursing home and instruct the staff or work directly with the residents.

☐ Community colleges or nearby universities usually offer pertinent courses in psychology, social work, gerontology, and various allied health fields that relate directly to the training of group leaders. Classes in group dynamics, aging, and psychology are particularly useful. Also, professionals from local mental health agencies will often volunteer their services to provide instruction in their respective disciplines.

☐ Religious denominations frequently have departments concerned with aging and its problems. Much of the material in these pastoral programs can be readily adapted for nursing home care, and various religious groups are invariably pleased to offer their help.

☐ Programs for the handicapped, such as Adventures in Movement (A.I.M.), usually provide training in dealing with the elderly and can be a valuable resource.

☐ Massage therapists can be invited to the nursing home to discuss issues about the body and emotions. (It is a worthwhile experience for group leaders themselves to receive a series of professional therapeutic massages in order to experience the feeling of true relaxation that comes with this method.)

☐ Art therapists and music therapists can usually be found in local colleges and universities.

☐ Professional musicians, especially older musicians, can often provide an understanding of how the experience of music can benefit residents.

In recruiting a cadre of teaching volunteers, it is important that the volunteer understands that the goal of the team is to involve, not to entertain. Therefore, in seeking and developing volunteers, look for someone who is not just a "do-gooder," but a person who is sensitive to the need for a richer and more fulfilling life for elders.

Problems Encountered by Group Leaders

Despite personal motivation and desire to enhance the lives of others, many problems arise which challenge even the strongest group leader. It is pertinent to consider briefly some typical problems:

☐ The staff of the nursing home who are not involved with your group activities may not understand your enthusiasm for your work and indeed may minimize your efforts.

☐ Because there is always so much to do in a nursing home, so little time, and never enough staff, it is not uncommon to experience difficulty in getting general staff members to cooperate in your program; for instance, in order for the group to function effectively, it is necessary to bring the residents to the group session in time and to bring them back to their rooms or to their next activity after the program. This, however, is often easier said than done, and personnel may not be available to assist your effort or may be occupied with other duties. Some members of the general staff may be skeptical about the value of your program and think you are overly idealistic in your goals. They may disparage the group program by considering it just fun and games.

☐ A feeling of resentment can develop if the group leader is relieved of certain other duties in order to lead the group. The staff may feel that they have to increase their workload to handle your normal responsibilities during the period of your group leadership.

These problems are of course annoying and can certainly interfere with the group's function and the group leader's enthusiasm. What can be done about these staff relations, and how can these problems be solved? The best method is to be patient while seeking opportunities to educate the individual members of the staff about the program, particularly those who are disdainful. The opportunities to discuss your programs with staff members may come in many ways; for example, a staff member may begin to see improvement in a resident and want to know what has been done, and what has happened. Or the staff may become aware that the residents look forward to attending the group and enjoy the group activities; again, they may inquire about this or about the fact that a particular resident is expressing himself or responding in new ways. In a somewhat different vein, staff members who have learned about the importance given to relaxation as practiced by the group may wish to participate in the relaxation program, which has a broad appeal to harried people. The main point is that the group leaders must make every opportunity to establish a cooperative relationship with every level of staff and try to involve them in some way in the group's program. Clearly, the more support from the staff for the program, the easier and more succesful the program will be. (An outline of the training program for the general staff follows this chapter.)

The Rewards of Being a Group Leader

In accepting the responsibilities of being a group leader and taking on the burden of training one's self in new disciplines, it is not unusual to weigh the effort required and the problems encountered against the anticipated benefits of this program. In our experience we find that the personal rewards of assuming this demanding role far exceed any disadvantages. The learning process itself is bene-ficial—many of the things you learn will become an integral part of your life style, such as exercises, diet, better communication, relaxation both at work and at home. The leader develops a greater understanding of emotions, of laughter, play and relaxation skills. Above all, perhaps, are the pleasure and personal satisfaction that come with an important job. The motivation, enthusiasm and approach to living that accompany this work will serve you well for the rest of your life.

Other than the personal rewards derived from this work, the group leader has the satisfaction of knowing this effort has an important and favorable influence on the lives of the residents of the institution. It is gratifying to observe residents learning new skills, developing confidence in expressing themselves, and showing greater

140

ability to reach out to others. Previously withdrawn residents may become motivated to enter rehabilitative programs and interrupt the downhill course of their lives.

Finally, a group program of this type has a beneficial effect on the entire institution, especially the general staff. It is not unusual in our experience for individual staff members, after being exposed to the group's goals and philosophies, to respond with increased self-responsibility and personal growth of their own. As a result, the staff may become more versatile and more satisfied with their jobs and with themselves. An institution with a satisfied staff provides a sense of community and serves to attract more residents.

Longevity Therapy:
The Relationship among Residents, Staff and Administration

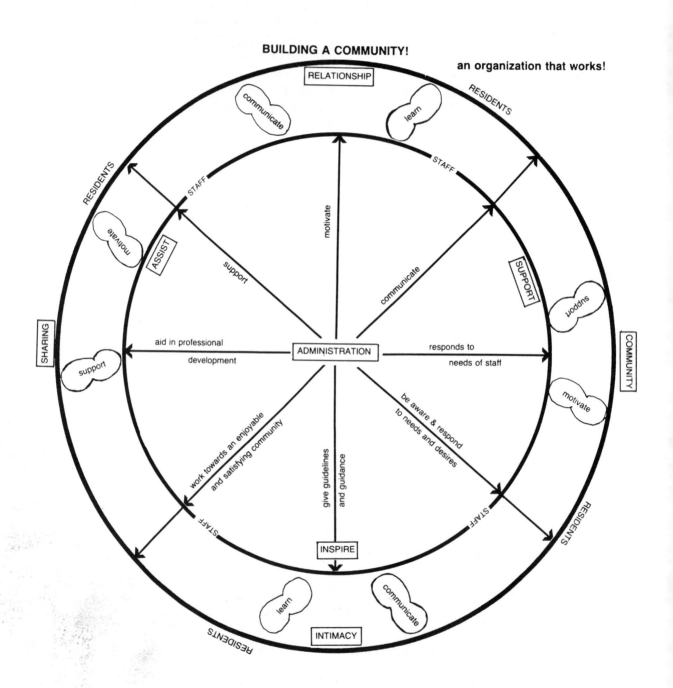

Nursing Home Staff Development Program

The Longevity Therapy staff, as mentioned, requires the cooperation and assistance of the general staff of the nursing home to achieve its goals. The nursing home staff, however, is often besieged with other duties and may not always be able to provide the help required. Moreover, there is sometimes a tendency for the general staff to minimize the importance of the specialized activities conducted by the Longevity Therapy group, viewing the activities as non-essential and in the "fun and games" category. As a result, the relationship between the nursing home staff and the Longevity Therapy staff may sometimes become strained, or at least trying, for both groups. For these reasons, it is important for both groups to participate in a development program designed to promote cooperation and to create a cohesive and caring environment for the residents and the staff.

The Development Program

We have found that these objectives can be accomplished through three means: frequent, small group staff-training programs; weekly resident and staff experiential group sessions; and individual staff consultations. The methods and conclusions described below are based on the results of an ongoing staff development project conducted by the senior members of the Longevity Therapy group.

One of the primary goals of this development program is to enhance job motivation and provide education for staff. This in turn helps to establish a pleasant institutional atmosphere that brings out the best in the residents.

Indeed, we believe that the existing negative image of nursing homes can be changed greatly by combining a milieu based on the true needs of the residents with deliberate planning, productive staff training and a functioning support system.

The details of the staff development program we employ are

outlined below. Included in these staff development sessions are members of the nursing, housekeeping, dietary and administrative staffs.

Group Staff Training Programs

Twice a week, members of the nursing home staff, especially the nursing staff, should meet jointly with representatives of the Longevity Therapy team to discuss a range of general issues concerning aging and the lives of older adults in general. Some of the areas that may be covered during these sessions are:

- ☐ Physical and emotional losses due to the aging process
- ☐ New residents' problems of adjustment to the nursing home
- ☐ How to apply verbal and nonverbal communication skills
- ☐ How to use motivational techniques
- ☐ Stress management methods for residents and staff
- ☐ The great importance of enhancing residents' self-image and self-esteem
- ☐ The value of Longevity Therapy activities such as movement, self-expression, play, music, in maintaining physical and emotional health.

Experiential Group Sessions

In order to help residents and staff communicate their thoughts and feelings and develop a closer bond of understanding, experiential group sessions should be conducted about every two weeks or so. The use of creative arts (music, art and poetry) provides a valuable means for sharing the wealth of experiences many individuals possess, but which are not readily apparent in a nursing home setting. Sharing these experiences through creative arts often leads to mutual respect and empathy.

Consultation

It is helpful to conduct a minimum of two meetings per month with the nursing home director and the various department heads. In this way all parties become aware of common problems, thereby allowing solutions to be formulated. Staff training, stress reduction, family issues and related topics should be offered to all nursing home staff through a series of one-hour workshops combined with individual consultation.

Staff Orientation

Before embarking on the program just outlined, nursing home staff members should be oriented to the concept of Longevity Therapy through a one-and-a-half hour lecture/workshop. This orientation session is meant to provide an overview of the goals of Longevity Therapy for the nursing home and to explain the processes and activities in which staff and residents participate. Staff orientation is usually conducted every two months to familiarize new staff members with the Longevity Therapy program.

The following material should be included in the orientation sessions:

Overview of the Longevity Therapy program

"You probably think old people just like to sit around, play bingo, watch soap operas, talk about how badly they feel, reminisce about the good old times and complain about the lousy new times. Don't you believe it! Elderly people enjoy loving, touching, learning, expressing their thoughts and feelings, laughing, joking, feeling sensual, hugging, kissing and creating new things."

Remember, above all, old people are able to grow mentally, emotionally, and spiritually until their last days.

Longevity Therapy focuses on the positive aspects of aging, helping individuals to accept themselves at this special stage of life. The program also allows the residents to feel more connected to others, to develop a positive sense of themselves, and to recognize a sense of purpose in their lives. These goals are accomplished by the use of many different techniques, including training in assertiveness, movement, methods of breathing, art activities, to name a few."

In order to provide emotional and psychological support to the residents, nursing home staff members must appreciate the problems of the elderly, and recognize how nursing home personnel can help resolve them. To this end, the following topics are suitable for discussion, learning and sharing during the twice weekly staff training session:

☐ The aging process and the associated emotional, physical and spiritual changes that accompany it
☐ Myths about aging
☐ Psychological and social implications of entering a nursing home
☐ Family dynamics and how to help the family cope with conflicting emotions arising from placing one of their members in a nursing home

- How families can improve the quality of the resident's life in the nursing home
- The importance of increasing and retaining self-esteem among the residents
- The importance of touch, movement and expression in the lives of the elderly
- Finding new meaning in life in later years
- The importance of communication between residents and staff.

In conducting these sessions, the leader should stress the idea that the underlying intent of the program is to provide the staff members with practical skills that can be used in their daily work and lives. While learning more about the residents and why they behave in certain ways, staff members discover more about themselves as well. Remember, we can help others only to the extent that we ourselves feel healthy—mentally, emotionally and spiritually. By improving the outlook of the residents as well as the staff itself, a nursing home community becomes a more enlivening and enjoyable place to be.

The Role of the Staff in Longevity Therapy

Staff members should appreciate the importance of their role in helping others. Indeed, staff members' interaction with the residents can often have a profound effect on the residents' lives. In effect, you the staff are their family and your attitude toward them goes a long way in determining how they respond. Your help is essential to make others appreciate the fundamental concept that every day is a new day for growth, love, appreciating life and being appreciated.

Although all health care personnel are taught to "take care" of the elderly, this help is often perceived in the sense of taking care of a pet—feeding, grooming and exercising. The staff must do more than "take care" of residents in this protective way: The object is not merely to "take care" but rather to relate to the residents as individuals and enjoy life with them. Such a relationship, in effect, completes a circle of energy and sharing—emotionally, physically and spiritually.

In this same regard, just as giving to others is one of the most enriching experiences a person can have, so is learning how to receive from others. Residents should be given the full opportunity to give of themselves, and the staff should be encouraged to receive gracefully the many treasures—often surprising treasures—the residents possess.

Some Myths About Aging

As noted in the Overview of Longevity Therapy, it is often assumed that old age is associated with the disappearance of all mental, physical and emotional ability. The common belief that elderly residents can do little more than watch soap operas or perform simple-minded tasks is *simply not true.* It is essential for the leader to reiterate this point during the orientation session. One way to bring home this idea is to review the following list:

Things That Do Not Change Throughout Life

- ☐ Interest in life, in staying active
- ☐ The need to feel connected with others; to be part of a group, family, or organization
- ☐ The need to work at something or perform tasks that represent one's self. (This can be an expressive hobby or a job; both tasks aid in the development of self-esteem.)
- ☐ Interest in sexuality
- ☐ The need for relationships and intimacy
- ☐ The need to communicate, to express one's feelings and thoughts, whether nonverbally through the arts, or verbally in conversation.
- ☐ Sensuality
- ☐ The need to learn and discover new things
- ☐ The sense of the timelessness and immortality of self: "The body grows old, not the person."
- ☐ The enjoyment of laughter
- ☐ The enjoyment of good food, good company, and pleasant suroundings
- ☐ The need to be productive and have a sense of purpose in life
- ☐ The need to touch and be touched by others—physically, emotionally and spiritually
- ☐ The need to love and be loved.

Definition of An Elder

An appropriate way to end the orientation sessions is to read and discuss "Definition of An Elder" by Barry Barkin of the Live Oak Institute, Oakland, California.*

> *"An Elder is a person who is still growing, still a learner, still with potential, and whose life continues to have within it promise for and connection to, the future. An Elder is still in pursuit of happiness, joy and pleasure, and his or her birthright to these remains intact. Moreover, an Elder is a person who deserves respect and honor and whose work it is to synthesize from long-life experience and formulate this into a legacy for future generations."*

---

*Wall-size posters of "Definitions of An Elder" are available from the Live Oak Living Center, Greenridge Heights, 2150 Pyramid Drive, El Sobrante, California 94803.

Ongoing Staff Development Sessions

Objectives

The staff development program has many different goals, which can be broadly classified under the following headings:

- ☐ To help you do your job most effectively and to enjoy your work
- ☐ To help residents by assessing their needs, by communicating with them, and by supporting them in their daily lives
- ☐ To learn something about yourself and how you can feel better physically, emotionally and spiritually using Longevity Therapy techniques
- ☐ To make the nursing home a happy and enjoyable community for residents and staff.

The Instructional Program

The sessions are held twice weekly for about 45 minutes each. The Longevity Therapy staff should be available for individual meetings as well as to discuss problems, staff interests, and to exchange ideas. The ongoing program usually lasts for three months or longer and involves members of the nursing, housekeeping, dietary and administrative staffs.

These training sessions are designed to cover four major areas:

- ☐ **Gerontological information** Physical and psychosocial changes in aging; myths of aging
- ☐ **Community building** Promoting a support network among staff and residents
- ☐ **Individual potential** Using the job as a tool for self-development, learning, and pleasure
- ☐ **Communication and motivational skills** Enhancing the staff's abilities to *(a)* communicate effectively and *(b)* encourage and motivate residents to achieve optimum independence.

Each session is dedicated to a particular theme (for example, "Emotional Aspects of Aging"). An outline and description of suggested formats for the first eight training sessions follows. Training sessions should be designed to fit the needs of particular personnel.

Session 1

Subject   **Residents' transition to life in a nursing home**

Introduction   Make a list of ten things most valuable in life to you. Now cross off two of them. Consider how difficult it is to lose just two things that are valuable to you. Can you imagine the loss residents feel when they must leave their customary surroundings and move into a nursing home?

Discussion   Ask the staff to share stories they know about transitions to a nursing home. Point out the losses the residents have endured and consider how these losses affect attitudes and behavior.

Lead staff in a discussion of what can be done to help residents in this difficult transition and adjustment.

Have the staff discuss experiences of their successes with residents who have had difficulty in adjusting to nursing home life.

Session 2

Subject   **Staff involvement in a nursing home setting**

Introduction   How to make a nursing home a true home? What contributions can we make and do we make to the patients' lives every day? Let's just dream a little. Take a minute and close your eyes. Take a deep breath, let your mind create an image of the nursing home. What do you like about this nursing home? How would you make it a better place? What particular feelings, attitudes, relationships, etc. would you like to find here? How would you really want this nursing home to be?

Discussion	Let the staff discuss the issues/images that they envisioned. Make a list. Identify things they can immediately begin to work on. Discuss what it takes to build a supportive, loving community consisting of staff members and patients. Examine the chart "Building a Community" (see next page) and review the ingredients for working together. These ingredients are to support, motivate, communicate and learn from each other and the patients. By utilizing these four ingredients you build relationships, intimacy, and a sense of community.

Session 3

Subject	**Vision and hearing loss: How to help residents adapt**
Introduction	Show the filmstrip, "Vision and Hearing Changes," produced by (and available from) the University of Michigan.
Discussion	Have staff discuss residents who have been able to adapt to their limitations. Explore what positive aspects of the residents' abilities have helped them adapt. Talk about what staff can do to inspire other residents to adjust more positively to living with their handicaps.

Session 4

Subject	**The process of aging**
Introduction	Ask staff to make a list of their own fears and expectations in growing older. Have the group share their responses.

Discussion

How do your own feelings about aging affect your work with older people?

Do you have many preconceived notions of what older people are going through?

Do you believe that elderly people can learn new things? What would it take for them to learn? How can they discover their strengths while they are confronting their weaknesses?

Lead a discussion on the topic of old age as a special time for growth and learning (*see* Philosophy in Section One). Point out that old age is a time for self-discovery according to Carl Jung and many Eastern cultures.

Session 5

Subject

Family involvement

Introduction

Present a family situation involving a resident in the nursing home and help the staff discuss the situation. Help them identify the issues mentioned below and their roles in that situation.

Discussion

Important points to include:

☐ Family's sense of guilt which can manifest as demanding behavior toward staff
☐ Resident's sense of loss of family, which can lead to depression, dependent behavior, and frustration
☐ What can families do to help?
☐ How can staff help families deal more effectively with the resident?

Session 6

Subject	**Communication**
Introduction	One of the most important but neglected ways of helping another person is to communicate thoughtfully. Communication is giving and receiving on both the verbal and nonverbal level. Giving means expressing oneself. Receiving means listening. Understand that giving and receiving can be interchangeable. *Being a receptive listener is a true gift.*
Discussion	Develop a list of keys to thoughtful communication. Introduce the following ideas:

☐ Listening without judgment
☐ Using the word "I" instead of "you" when expressing opinions or feelings
☐ Using eye contact and other nonverbal means (such as touch) to express acceptance of the speaker
☐ Distinguishing between assertiveness and aggressiveness
☐ Identifying the difference between clear communication and manipulative communication

Session 7

Subject	**Motivation**
Introduction	Ask the staff what motivates and inspires them in their daily lives.
Discussion	Focus on how staff can motivate residents.

☐ Notice even the smallest positive change in residents' attitudes, activities and behavior and acknowledge the change you have observed, praising the resident for his/her effort.

□ Inspire residents by demonstrating a respect and appreciation for what the resident has accomplished in life.
□ Help each resident function as independently as possible. Provide the opportunity for them to make independent choices.

Session 8

Subject   **Emotional care of residents**

Introduction   Emotional care is a reciprocal process. As we care for the resident we also derive emotional support and nurturing for ourselves. It is vital to continue to clarify our own needs and feelings as staff members and health care workers as we attempt to serve others.

Discussion   Some issues to consider:

□ How to provide a nurturing environment for the resident
□ What are the components of emotional care (psychological and social)?
□ What may prevent you from paying attention to the emotional needs of a patient?
□ Why the staff may feel anger, fear and frustration in dealing with the residents, families, the administration, and other staff members
□ How to meet this challenge and become more effective in offering emotional care to the residents.

The Foundations of Longevity Therapy:
Personal Reflections

—Bobbie R. Graubarth-Szyller

My involvement in working with elders in long-term care began in 1960, when my father was placed in a nursing home. In my daily visits to him, I found that he was given good custodial care, but it was on a typical medical/hospital basis. The disease was attended, but not the human being.

I visited with other residents, going from room to room. Whenever I asked the right questions, most residents became individuals, with spirit in their voices and in their eyes. How did I come up with the right questions? Partially from intuition, but mostly I listened for positive key words. With these words I could identify their strengths and focus on positive stories and expressions. When residents were listened to, something wonderful happened. Their stories transcended their depression and apathy. I learned that it was our interaction *at that moment* that was important.

I realized that human potential was largely being ignored in institutions, but that given the opportunity it could flourish. The whole person needed attending. The resident was not simply a heart patient, or a fracture patient with limitations, but an individual whose strengths, if we could identify and encourage them, could be put to use.

I knew that some day I wanted to work with elders in long-term care.

During the next few years, I began to look at my life more closely. I started by working on changing some of my ideas about myself—how I responded to life, work, family, relationships. I wanted to develop my intuition and create a life with more harmony. I searched for answers. I found people who became my teachers and mentors, who would influence my thinking and development profoundly in the future.

It was through yoga classes that I discovered more freedom with my body. Until then, because of arthritis, I was unable to get up in the morning without crawling out of bed backwards, on my knees. After daily stretching and practicing yoga *asanas* (exercise), I learned an important lesson: to function better I had to assume the responsibility myself. I had more vitality and complained less. Little wonder that the first method I was to use in a long-term care facility was yoga; I could convincingly encourage others that the exercises worked!

Along the same line, I learned from a Bio-Energetics trainer therapeutic movement techniques to express feelings through words combined with exercises. Designed by Dr. Alexander Lowen, these exercises allow the body to flow with energy, eliminating fatigue and inertia. Moreover, the exercises are a technique for understanding the personality in terms of the body, enhancing many aspects of personality by releasing and mobilizing energy ordinarily bound up by muscular tension. Also, one's capacity to experience pleasure is increased.

Yoga and Bio-Energetics taught me about relaxation and release of tension in my body. I also began to learn about body massage and experienced the bodily changes that can take place with touch.

In 1975 I attended a Wellness Seminar at the University of Michigan. "Wellness" was a new concept to me. I was only beginning to understand the real difference between health and sickness. Many authors—doctors, teachers and therapists—presented papers. I attended Dr. Carl Symington's lecture based on his book *Getting Well Again*. His stories about his cancer patients and his approach to their wellness were fascinating. He used traditional medications, but added components of good nutrition (live food, not canned or treated with chemicals), laughter, play, humor and visualization techniques. I learned that visualization allows one to relax and become receptive to new ideas and feelings, encouraging a more positive self-image and new ways of maintaining health. For example, in cancer treatment a person uses an image, or imagination, to gobble up the cancer by visualizing a hungry Pac-Man eating the pain. Dr. Symington reported that his patients were able to eliminate pain and achieve a fuller, higher quality life than before. He believes that visualization is a modality of self-help that can mobilize the immune system and our internal healing capabilities.

I also attended a lecture given by Richard Alpert, also known as Baba Ram Dass, a spiritual teacher and a former professor of psychology at Harvard University. I had no idea how profound an effect his teaching would have on me. He had just written a book, *Be Here Now,* whose philosophy I would carry into my life and, later, into my work. *Be Here Now* advocates not holding onto the past nor worrying about the future, but being aware of and appreciating the present. This was a new and important idea for me. I subsequently studied with him at the University of Florida, where he taught yogic breathing and meditation and discussed spiritual growth in each stage of ife. He demonstrated techniques for silencing the mind and for expressing negative thoughts and emotions (anger, jealousy, rage, fear) that seem to stay with us unless asked to leave. We used a simple ritual of writing a negative thought on a piece of paper and throwing it into a bonfire. I learned that one could throw away uselss, negative concepts that kept the body/mind from being a finely tuned instrument.

After these experiences I felt I was ready to start working in long-term care. I continued my development by taking a summer course at the Institute of Gerontology at the University of Michigan, where I received more direction in creating a healthy environment in a long-term care setting. Dorothy Coons, the director, saw me as a student who was a "human blotter," I was so eager. The fact is that I was opening my mind, I truly wanted to learn. When you are curious and are really interested in knowing something, learning becomes easier. Not only did I experience fewer mental barriers, but also a flow of energy, creativity and intuition entered the learning process.

A few years later I asked the Institute of Gerontology to help me design Longevity Therapy into a teaching model and received input from a team of educators, psychologists, group planners and health professionals. The end product was a 17-session curriculum. Dorothy Coons continues to give me support and encouragement, and I consider her to be an important contributor to my work and to the field of gerontology.

I also took courses in sociology, psychology, and the physiology of aging at the Scripps Howard Gerontological Institute at Miami University, Oxford, Ohio. I became certified as an A.I.M. (Adventures in Movement) instructor for the handicapped. A.I.M. taught me methods of leading movement exercise for handicapped children, and I began to apply those methods with older people. As a consequence, A.I.M. teachers began to include the elderly in their curriculum.

I continued studies in Eastern philosophy when a friend, Kitty Chi, married a Chinese man, a teacher of Taoism. I began to read the *Tao Te Ching.* I learned Tai Chi (Tai Chi Ch'uan), the movement that expresses Taoist philosophy, which is based on the interplay of balance and strength. I learned that strength can come from nonmovement—a particularly good lesson for active people! I became a regular student of Tai Chi, a slow, graceful exercise, and soon was taking this movement into nursing homes. Because Tai Chi works to establish balance (internally and externally), it can be used to address one of the biggest fears in aging, that of falling. It is very hard to keep a positive attitude when one falls. It is a shock, an imbalance. To overcome shock and promote mending, balance needs to be present in body, mind and spirit. Tai Chi helps me to give balance in all three. Even if the body begins to fail, mind and spirit can remain in balance.

In 1979 I met one of my finest teachers and inspirations, Gay Gaer Luce, at that time director of SAGE (Senior Actualization and Growth Explorations). I had heard about this California-based group for many years and knew they were expanding the frontiers of humanistic gerontology. I took a seminar from Gay Luce, after several years of using the methods I developed. She introduced me to the philosophy of Rinpoche, who said "The first part of life is for learning; the second part of life is for service; the third part of life is for self."

I read that in the East, elders looked forward to retirement and wanted time to develop themselves. This statement was proof of what I had understood about the Eastern philosophy of aging. Why was it so different from American myths of aging? In our country, retirement means "over the hill." When I read Gay Luce's *Your Second Life,* I further saw how different old age can be. I became convinced that growth can occur at eighty as well as at eight.

Finally, I kept investigating the best nursing home programs in the country, looking for teachers and visionaries. I found one in Barry Barkin, designer and director of the Live Oak Project. One of his approaches to long-term care is to build a community within a nursing home, establishing daily community meetings at which discussions of events, stories and song are used to form a structure of consciousnes for staff and residents. The stronger resident helps the less strong. The community has a very supportive, loving environment. His Elder Poster should be in every nursing home. He gives dignity to the word "Elder."

At the SAGE training program I met Julie Padgett. She had just completed a master's degree program in social work with a certificate in gerontology at the University of Michigan. She too was strongly attracted to the concepts and hope of the new alternatives available to older people. When she decided to return to her hometown of New Orleans, where I was living, we decided to work together.

We met Jules Weiss several years into our development of this program. His strong concern for spiritual development and his great sense of humor added to our lives. He is a good friend whose own work is an important contribution to expressive therapy.

These were the foundations of Longevity Therapy.

The diagrams shown here and on the opposite page summarize (1) the role changes that accompany aging, and (2) the manner in which these changes can be altered by intervention in the form of Longevity Therapy.

The Role Change Spiral

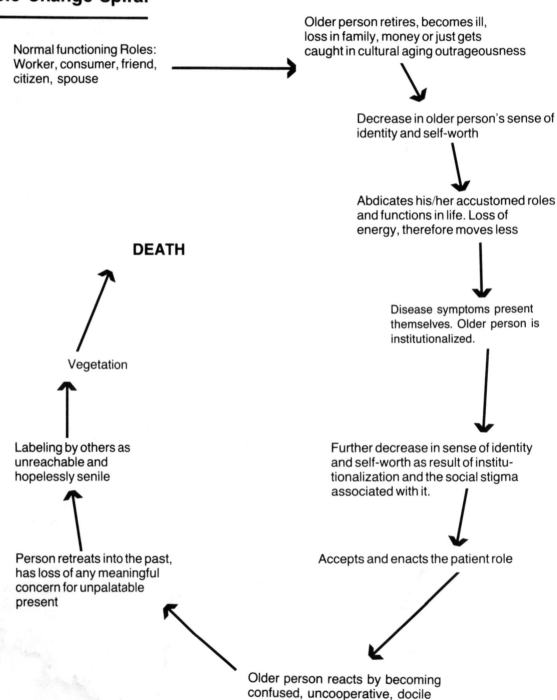

Normal functioning Roles: Worker, consumer, friend, citizen, spouse

Older person retires, becomes ill, loss in family, money or just gets caught in cultural aging outrageousness

Decrease in older person's sense of identity and self-worth

Abdicates his/her accustomed roles and functions in life. Loss of energy, therefore moves less

Disease symptoms present themselves. Older person is institutionalized.

Further decrease in sense of identity and self-worth as result of institutionalization and the social stigma associated with it.

Accepts and enacts the patient role

Older person reacts by becoming confused, uncooperative, docile or regressed

Person retreats into the past, has loss of any meaningful concern for unpalatable present

Labeling by others as unreachable and hopelessly senile

Vegetation

DEATH

Reversal of the Role Change Spiral

OLDER PERSON retires
Becomes ill
Loss in family
Loss of money or just
gets caught in
Cultural Aging Outrageousness

⟶

Decrease in Older Person's
sense of identity and self-worth

Loss of energy; therefore
moves less

Disease symptoms
present themselves

**HEALTH MAINTENANCE THROUGH
PERSONAL RESPONSIBILITY**

INTERVENTION MUST OCCUR AT THIS
POINT OR PREFERABLY BEFORE.

Trust relationship with
teacher, with movement, vitality,
philosophy, breathing, touching
techniques

Healthy Philosophy Reinforced
on a regular basis, Trust
Relationship expanding to
Love of Self

Interaction with peer group, releasing
and sharing problems thru group

Expression added to movement through
games, toning, art

161

Suggested Reading

Adventures in Movement for the Handicapped. 943 Danbury Road, Dayton, Ohio.

Ballantine, Rudolph M. *Joints and Glands Exercises.* Honesdale, PA: Himalayan International Institute, 1978.

Berkus, R. *Appearances.* Encino, CA: Red Rose Press, 1984.

Birren, J. E. and R. B. Sloane (eds). *Handbook of Mental Health and Aging.* Englewood Cliffs, NJ: Prentice-Hall, 1980.

Bliss, Shepherd. *The New Holistic Health Handbook: Living Well in a New Age.* Lexington, MA: Stephen Green Press, 1985.

Bonny, Helen. *Music and Your Mind.* New York: Harper and Row, 1973.

Brenner, Paul. *Health Is A Question of Balance.* New York: DeVross Publishers, 1982.

Brown, Mollie (ed.). *Readings in Gerontology.* St. Louis: C. V. Mosby Co., 1978.

Burnside, Irene. *Working with the Elderly: Group Process & Techniques.* North Scituate, MA: Duxbury Press, 1978.

Butler, R. and H. Gleason. *Productive Aging.* New York: Springer, 1985.

Butler, R. and M. Lewis. *Aging and Mental Health: Positive Psychological Approaches.* St. Louis: C. V. Mosby Co., 1977.

Christenson, Alice and David Rankin. *Easy Does it Yoga.* Cleveland Heights, OH: Saraswati Studio, 1976.

Comfort, Alex. *A Good Age.* New York: Crown, 1976.

Coons, Dorothy, L. Metzelaar, A. Robinson, B. Spencer. *A Better Life.* Columbus, OH: The Source, 1986.

Cousins, Norman. *Anatomy of An Illness.* New York: Norton, 1979.

_____ *Human Options.* New York: Norton, 1984.

Delaney, Gayle, *Living Your Dreams.* New York: Harper and Row, 1979.

De Vries, Herbert. *Vigor Regained.* Englewood Cliffs, NJ: Prentice-Hall, 1974.

Doress, P. and D. Siegal. *Ourselves, Growing Older.* New York: Simon and Schuster, 1987.

Doty, Leilani. *Communication and Assertion Skills for Older Persons.* Washington, D.C.: Hemisphere Publishing Corp., 1987.

Dychtwald, Kenneth. *Bodymind.* New York: Jove, 1977.

_____ *Age Wave.* Los Angeles: Jeremy Tarcher, 1989.

Euster, Gerald L. "A sysem of groups in institutions for the aged." *Social Casework.* 52:523-39 (Nov.), 1971.

Fallcreek, S., et al. *Health Promotion and Aging: A National Directory of Selected Programs,* Washington, DC, U.S. Administration of Aging, 1986.

Fallcreek, S. and M. Mettler. *A Healthy Old Age: A Sourcebook for Health Promotion with Older Adults.* Washington, DC: Dept. of Health and Human Services, Administration on Aging, 1984.

Fleshman, Bob. *The Arts in Therapy.* Chicago, IL: Nelson-Hall, 1981.

Flugelman, Andrew (ed). *New Games.* New York: Doubleday, Dolphin, 1976.

Garfield, Charles. *The Psychosocial Care of the Aging Patient.* New York: McGraw-Hill, 1978.

Gawain, Shakti. *Creative Visualization.* San Rafael, CA: Whatever Publishing, 1978.

_____ *Living in the Light.* San Rafael, CA: Whatever Publishing, 1986.

Geba, Bruno. *Vitality Training for Older Adults.* New York: Random House, 1974.

Goldwasser, A. N. et al. "Cognitive, affective and behavioral effects of reminiscence group therapy on demented elderly." *International Journal of Aging and Human Development* 25(3):209-222, 1987.

Greene, Roberta R. *Social Work with the Aged and Their Families.* Hawthorne, NY: Aldine de Gruyter, 1986.

Gross, R., et al. *The New Old: Struggle for a Decent Aging.* New York: Anchor Books, 1978.

Halpern, Steven, with Louis Savory. *Sound Health: The Music and Sounds that Make Us Whole.* San Francisco: Harper and Row, 1985.

Hamblin, K. *Mime: a Playbook of Silent Fantasy.* Garden City, NY: Doubleday, 1978.

Hay, Louise L., *You Can Heal Your Life.* Santa Monica, CA: 1984.

Herr, John J. and John H. Weakland. *Counseling Elders and Their Families.* New York: Springer, 1979.

Houston, Jean. *The Possible Human.* Los Angeles: J. P. Tarcher, 1982.

Hunag, Al Chung Liang. *Embrace Tiger, Return to Mountain.* New York: Bantam, 1973.

Hurley, Olga. *Safe Therapeutic Exercise for the Frail Elderly: An Introduction.* Albany, NY: Center for the Study of Aging, 1988.

Ingersoll, B. and L. Goodman. "History comes alive: Facilitating reminiscence in a group of institutionalized elderly." *Journal of Gerontological Social Work* 2:No. 4 (Summer 1980): 305-320.

Johnson, Don. *The Protean Body.* New York: Harper Row, 1977.

Johnson, David, W. and Frank P. Johnson. *Joining Together: Group Theory and Group Skills.* Englewood Cliffs, NJ: Prentice Hall, 1982.

Jung, Carl G. *Psychological Reflections.* Princeton, NJ: Princeton University Press, 1973.

Kaminsky, Marc. *The Uses of Reminiscence: New Ways of Working with Older Adults.* New York: Haworth Press, 1984.

Keleman, S. *The Human Ground.* Palo Alto, CA: Science and Behavior Books. 1975.

Kemp, Donald W. et al. *Growing Wiser.* Boise, ID. Healthwise, 1986.

Keyes, Laurel. *Toning.* Santa Monica, CA: Devores and Co., 1973.

Koch, Kenneth. *I Never Told Anybody.* New York: Random House, 1977.

Kopp, Sheldon, *Even A Stone Can Be A Teacher: Learning and Growing From the Experiences of Everyday Life.* Los Angeles: Jeremy Tarcher. 1985.

Krieger, Dolores. *Therapeutic Touch.* New York: Prentice Hall, 1979.

Kübler-Ross, Elisabeth. *Death: The Final Stage of Growth.* Englewood Cliffs, NJ: Prentice Hall, 1975.

LaBorde, Genie. *Influencing with Integrity.* Palo Alto, CA: Science and Behavior Books. 1984.

Langer, Ellen and Judith Rodin. "The effects of choice and enhanced personal responsibility for the aged: A field experiment in an institutional setting." *Journal of Personality and Social Psychology* 34:2, 191-198, 1975.

LeBlanc, Donna. "Case studying the philosophy, integrity and emotional health of the elderly." *Educational Gerontology* 13(5):387-402, 1987.

Lingerman, Hal. *The Healing Energies of Music.* Wheaton, IL: Theosophical Publishing House, 1983.

Lowen, Alexander. *Bioenergetics.* New York: Penguin Books, 1980.

_____. *Pleasure: A Creative Approach to Life.* New York: Penguin, 1970.

Luce, Gay Gaer. *Your Second Life.* New York: Delacorte Press, 1979.

Mandel, Evelyn. *The Art of Aging.* Minneapolis, MN: Winston Press, 1981.

Maslow, A. *Toward a New Psychology of Being.* New York: Van Nostrand, 1968.

Montague, Ashley. *Touching.* New York: Harper and Row, 1971.

Myerhoff, B. *Number Our Days.* New York: Simon and Schuster, 1978.

Norris, Patricia, and Garrett Porter. *I Choose Life: The Dynamics of Visualization and Biofeedback.* Walpole, NH: Stillpoint Publishing, 1987.

Norton, Suza. *Yoga for People Over 50.* Old Greenwich, CT: Devin-Adair, 1977.

Nuernberger, Phil. *Freedom from Stress: A Holistic Approach.* Honesdale, PA: Himalayan International Institute, 1981.

Pease, Ruth. "Dependency and the double bind in the aged." *Journal of Gerontological Nursing.* 4:4 (July/Aug), 18-21, 1978.

Pelletier, Kenneth. *Mind as Healer, Mind as Slayer.* New York: Dell, 1977.

Penn, Cathy. "Promoting independence." *Journal of Gerontological Nursing.* 14(3):14-19, 1988.

Priddy, J. Michael, et al. "Overcoming learned helplessness in elderly clients: Skills training for service providers." *Educational Gerontology* 8:507-518, 1982.

Ram Dass. *Be Here Now.* New York: Crown Publishers, 1971.

_____, *The Only Dance There Is.* Garden City, NY: Anchor/Doubleday, 1974.

Ram Dass and P. Gorman. *How Can I Help?* New York: Alfred A. Knopf, 1985.

Rhyne, Janie. *Gestalt Art Experiences.* Monterey, CA: Brooks/Cole, 1973.

Richards, Marty, et al. *Understanding Families: A Guidebook for Trainers of Nursing Home Staff.* University of Washington, Pacific Northwest, Long-Term Care Center, 1984.

Ryan, Regina Sara and John W. Travis. *The Wellness Workbook.* Berkeley, CA: Ten Speed Press. 1981.

Samuels, Mike and Nancy Samuels. *Seeing with the Mind's Eye: The History, Techniques and Uses of Visualization.* New York: Random House, 1975.

Saxon, Sue and Mary Jean Etten. *Physical Change and Aging.* New York: Tiresias Press, 1978.

Sekuler, Robert and Randolph Blake. "Sensory underload." *Psychology Today* 21(12):48-51, 1987.

Siegel, Bernard. *Love, Medicine and Miracles*. New York: Harper and Row, 1986.

Selye, Hans. *The Stress of Life*. New York: McGraw-Hill, 1956.

Sheehy, Gail. *Passages*. New York: E.P. Dutton, 1976.

Sherman, Edmund. "Reminiscence groups for community elderly." *The Gerontologist* 27(5):569-572, 1987.

Simonton, Carl and Stephanie Matthews Simonton. *Getting Well Again*. Los Angeles: Jeremy Tarcher, 1978.

Sri Swami Rama. *Exercise Without Movement: Yoga*. Honesdale, PA: Himalayan International Institue, 1984.

St. Pierre, Jeanne et al. "Late life depression: a guide for assessment." *Journal of Gerontological Nursing* 12(7):4-10. 1986.

Weisburg, N. and R. Wilder. *Creater Arts With Elder Adults: A Sourcebook*. New York: Human Science Press, 1984.

Weiss, Jules. *Expressive Therapy with Elders and the Disabled: Touching the Heart of Life*. New York: Haworth Press, 1984.

Wetzel, Janice Wood. "Interventions with the depressed elderly in institutions." *Social Casework*. April 1980:234-239.

Wu, John. *Lao Tzu*. New York: St. John University Press, 1977.

Zi, Nancy, *The Art of Breathing: 30 Simple Exercises for Improving Your Performance and Wellbeing*. San Francisco: Bantam Books, 1986.

Notes